YOUTH
SPORTS
INJURIES

◆

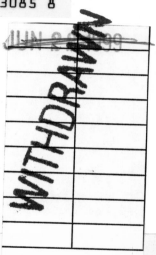

YOUTH

A Medical Handbook

SPORTS

for Parents and Coaches

INJURIES

♦

JOHN F. DUFF, M.D.

COLLIER BOOKS
Macmillan Publishing Company
New York

Maxwell Macmillan Canada
Toronto

Maxwell Macmillan International
New York   Oxford   Singapore   Sydney

Copyright © 1992 by John F. Duff
Illustrations © 1992 by Carol L. Reid

Collier Books   Maxwell Macmillan Canada, Inc.
Macmillan Publishing Company   1200 Eglinton Avenue East
866 Third Avenue   Suite 200
New York, NY 10022   Don Mills, Ontario M3C 3N1

Macmillan Publishing Company is part of the Maxwell Communication Group of Companies.

Library of Congress Cataloging-in-Publication Data
Duff, John F.
    Youth sports injuries : a medical handbook for parents and coaches
    John F. Duff ; illustrations by Carol L. Reid
        p.   cm.
    Includes index.
    ISBN 0-02-013691-9
    1. Pediatric sports medicine. 2. Sports for children—Accidents
    and injuries. I. Title.
    RC1218.C45D84   1992
    617.1'027—dc20   91-37789
                    CIP

Macmillan books are available at special discounts for bulk purchases for sales promotions, premiums, fund-raising, or educational use. For details, contact:

Special Sales Director
Macmillan Publishing Company
866 Third Avenue
New York, NY 10022

FIRST COLLIER BOOKS EDITION 1992

10 9 8 7 6 5 4 3 2 1

Printed in the United States of America

DESIGN BY LAURA HOUGH

This book is dedicated to Estamarie, my wife,

and to our eight children:

Kathleen, John, Cynthia, Christopher,

Elizabeth, Julia, Gregory,

and Mark.

◆

Contents

◆

Acknowledgments

◆

My indebtedness to Peter C. Reid, my writer/editor, is immeasurable. His writing expertise, combined with his energy and patience, developed my manuscript into an organized, readable reference for parents and coaches. I am grateful as well for the outstanding illustrations by Carol L. Reid, his wife.

There are several other major players without whose support my book would not have become a reality: Jeanine Bucek and Nancy Cooperman, my editors at Macmillan; Patricia C. Haskell, my agent; Laurie Pendleton, my secretary for seventeen years; Daniel Hanley, M.D., my mentor; William Sabin, my editor-coach; Fred Allman, M.D. and Paul Grace, athletic trainer, for their continued encouragement as the book evolved.

My sincere appreciation goes to the many parents, coaches, and professionals who read and critiqued the manuscript as it developed. These include Frank and Diane Agostino; Tenley Albright, M.D.; Joseph Arena, M.D.; Henry Banks, M.D.; Robert Cantu, M.D.; Harry Carpenter, M.D., and Vickie Carpenter; Andrew Clausen; Earl Cook; Daniel and Linda Curtis; Joseph Delansky; Mary Duff; Blair Filler, M.D.; William Gaine; Joseph Geike, Ph.D.; Rita Glassman; Robert Glabicky; Kelly Jefferson; John and Nancy Jones; John Kazes, M.D.; Sally Knapp, R.D.; Martin Korn, M.D.;

Gary Larabee; Richard McKallagut; Diane McKay; Michael Lovett, R.P.T.; Otto and Constance Moulton; Rosemary Baker, R.N.; Theresa Nyland; Rodney Pendleton; Maureen Pickard, R.N.; Robert Provost, M.D.; Walter Sargent, A.D.; Henry Sheldon; David St. Pierre, M.D.; Jon and Donna Tiplady; Paul Vinger, M.D.; E. K. Wallace, M.D.; and Douglas Wood, A.D.

I am also grateful to all the young athletes, their parents, and their coaches who contributed to the experience that made this book possible. The following experts gave me a strong vote of confidence when I first conceived this book: Robert Beaton; Kenneth Clarke, Ph.D.; Nathaniel Mac-Donald, M.D.; and Bertram Holland, M.D.

Finally, I must acknowledge my father, Paul H. Duff, M.D. (1894–1986), to whom I am indebted for the example he set as a physician. He was my guiding light.

Introduction

◆

Imagine yourself in the following situations:

- You are sitting in the bleachers watching your nine-year-old Barbara play in a youth soccer game. As she and two other girls converge on the ball, an opposing player accidentally kicks Barbara squarely on the shin. She falls to the ground and rolls onto her back, holding her leg as she screams in agony. By the time you reach the sidelines, the coach has carried her off the field, placed her on the bench, and is applying an ice pack. Your daughter is crying so hard you can barely hear the coach tell you not to worry.

  Should you insist that she be taken directly to the hospital?

- Your sixteen-year-old Robert comes home from lacrosse practice an hour later than usual. When you ask where he has been, he explains, "I really got my bell rung." Another player's stick had hit him in the head severely enough for the coach to take him out of the game and make him rest a while to be sure he was all right before he went home. He was not unconscious at any time. "Tell your mom or dad what happened," the coach had insisted. Robert says he is fine, despite having a severe headache.

Should you contact your physician? Go to the emergency room right away? Or wait to see how Robert is in the morning?

- The school nurse calls to say that your seven-year-old Wendy had an accident in gymnastics. "Wendy fell quite hard on her shoulder from the balance beam," the nurse explains. "Her arm went dead for several minutes and she had some pain. I think she'll need some ice and maybe some aspirin."
   Would you be satisfied that the nurse's advice was sufficient?

- Your Larry, aged fifteen, comes home from Babe Ruth League baseball practice with a swollen and bruised wrist. This all-star player slid into second base with his arm outstretched and landed on his wrist. "Gee," he says, "I sprained my wrist. Guess I can't do my math homework." "Guess you can't hold a spoon to eat ice cream tonight either," you respond. "Hey," he says, "the pain just went away!"
   Is this a simple sprain or should Larry see a doctor for this injury?

- You are proudly watching your seventeen-year-old high-schooler Bruce as he moves in for a solid hit on the opposing ball carrier in a big football game. Just as Bruce cuts to the right, he suddenly falls down. His knee has given out. His teammates and the trainer help him off the field and apply ice and an Ace elastic bandage. His knee begins to swell immediately and he has considerable pain. Even so, the stoic young player talks of getting his knee taped so that he can finish the game.
   Should you be arranging to take Bruce directly to the emergency room?

Five sports injuries. Five decisions that must be made by concerned parents. Would you be prepared to make the correct decisions? Most parents asked this question would have to say no. They are ill-equipped to determine what medical care should be given to their injured children and how immediately it should be given.

What compounds the problem is that some sports injuries aren't as serious as they appear, while others may seem innocuous but in fact can be severe and even life threatening. Let's look at the five injuries just described:

- *Barbara.* In a direct kick to the shinbone, the pain is almost always worse than the injury. Chances are that with a few minutes of rest, an ice pack, and a wrap over the bruise, your daughter could be right back in the game, a little sore but going full speed ahead.

- *Robert.* After being hit in the head, your youngster appears to be well, but in fact he could be carrying a time bomb. The blow may have produced a clot of blood on the brain. With certain head injuries there may be no complaints and no findings to indicate the severity of the injury, initially or even over a period of time. But should a clot expand in the brain before it is discovered, it could be fatal. *All head injuries should be investigated by a doctor immediately.*

- *Wendy.* The "dead arm" is usually not serious for a seven-year-old. However, if the pain does not subside and the arm motion return quickly, a "buckle fracture" of the shoulder may have occurred. Although not serious, it must be properly diagnosed and treated within a few days of the injury.

- *Larry.* Larry's "sprained wrist" is another potentially tragic situation. *An apparent sprained wrist should always be considered a fractured navicular bone until proven otherwise.* If it is a fracture and is not treated, it can severely impair the wrist and cause disabling arthritis in later life. Because the first X rays may be negative, it is essential to X-ray the wrist immediately *and two weeks later,* followed by a bone scan should there be any doubt about the diagnosis.

• *Bruce.* Bruce's injured knee should be treated promptly. While this twist of the knee may at first appear to be a simple strain, it is probably a tear of the anterior cruciate ligament—a serious knee injury. Early care of this injury by an expert is critical.

These might be your kids. If they're not active in sports now, they probably will be when they're old enough. Today, the world is experiencing a remarkable boom in competitive sports, and youth sports are a big part of that boom. Almost every town and city in the United States now has organized sports activities for young people: Little League baseball, Pop Warner football, soccer, gymnastics, basketball, swimming, and others. Individual sports like figure skating, diving, tennis, bowling, rock-climbing, and fencing are also thriving amongst children. The average high-school athletic program now offers twenty-six different sports for boys and girls. As of 1991, there were more than twenty million youngsters active in sports in the United States.

That's a lot of kids. And it means a lot of injuries. Injuries during the growing years can have a significant impact on physical and emotional development. A good percentage leave permanent disabilities of varying severity. Psychologically, these injuries can be debilitating and demoralizing (although sometimes the experience of being injured can build self-confidence and maturity).

◆   **Why This Book?**

Over more than thirty years of treating youngsters with sports injuries I have made notes on all the things parents should know—*but don't know*—that could help them to prevent and minimize these injuries. The result is this book. Its aims are:

• To give you quick and easy reference to simple, understandable explanations of each specific type of sports injury (including helpful illustrations)

- To tell you what treatment is appropriate for a specific injury and what immediate action you should take when your child arrives home
- To help you to assess the risks of a given sport in which your youngster may want to participate (or already is participating) and to promote safety in that sport
- To give you a clear picture of what kinds of injuries may be involved in that sport—and their long-term consequences
- To explain good-quality care on the field, in the locker room, and in the medical office—so that you can make sure your child gets it
- To help you deal effectively with the coach, the trainer, the school nurse, the emergency medical technician, the therapist, the family physician, the sports medical specialist, and anyone else who may be involved in the care of your child's sports injury
- To help you evaluate a coach's recommendation or physician's advice on taking care of your child's sports injury
- To guide you in selecting a qualified sports medicine physician
- To help you understand the psychological impact of an injury on your youngster—and deal with that impact effectively
- To tell you how to make sure that your injured child does not return to active competition too early

◆ More Help

You will find additional features in back of the book that can help you become an expert on youth sports injuries:

Medical Terms: A Glossary
Locker Room Jargon: A Glossary
Resources on Sports Injuries and Safety
Resources on Specific Sports
Resources on Young Athletes with Disabilities
Resources on Coaching Education
Suggested Readings

◆   **The Bottom Line**

This book is designed to be used again and again. I firmly believe that if you and parents like you know what sports medical experts know, the whole sports injury picture would improve dramatically overnight. May this knowledge keep your young athletes healthy through their growing years so they can enjoy participating in sports over their whole lives.

PART I

The Values and Risks of Sports for Your Child

◆

1

How Safe Are Youth Sports Today?

◆

"What are the chances my child will be hurt playing sports?"

Are there any parents of sports-active boys and girls who don't have this question on their minds? Certainly not many. But for the most part, they just cross their fingers and hope that "nothing happens."

That's a precarious hope. One third of U.S. children who participate in sports suffer some kind of injury requiring attention from parents, physicians, or both. But there's a lot that parents *can* do besides crossing their fingers. Getting actively involved, dealing knowledgeably with your children's sports injuries, and working to make sports safer can help substantially to reduce the number of serious injuries with lasting effects.

With more and more children in competitive sports at younger and younger ages youth sports injuries present a growing problem that must be taken seriously. The National Athletic Trainers Association estimates that in 1990 at least one million high-school athletes suffered at least one sports injury. More than twenty thousand of these injuries required surgery.

These are just impersonal statistics. But they represent personal, painful, and sometimes permanent injuries. In your own neighborhood you probably often hear about such injuries. What happened to Greg? He sprained his ankle sliding into second base. What happened to Julie? She twisted her knee dismounting from her horse. What happened to Otis? He broke his thumb playing football.

Hearing about such injuries should raise some important questions in your mind:

- Are youth sports as safe as they can be?
- Are youth sports programs sufficiently dedicated to safety?
- How serious are sports injuries in general?
- What are the most common injuries in specific sports?
- Which sports tend to have the most serious injuries?

We'll deal with these questions in this section.

But first, you must face the fact that *there is no such thing as an injury-free sport.* Risks of injury exist in every sport. You must balance these risks against the benefits to be gained from the sport.

◆ ARE YOUTH SPORTS AS SAFE AS THEY CAN BE?

The answer is no, youth sports are not as safe as they can be. Good progress has been made in improving safety,

---

What Are Youth Sports?

Three major types of youth sports activities will be discussed throughout this book:
- Youth-League Sports: *Organized nonschool team sports for youngsters who are generally under the age of eighteen.*
- Individual Sports: *Sports in which solo performance is what counts rather than team play.*
- High-School Sports: *Sports programs for high-school students*

but there is much more that can be done to reduce the number and severity of injuries. Recommendations are given throughout this book.

Youth sports safety is getting more and more attention throughout the world. Sports medical meetings are crammed with discussions of prevention, while national youth sports organizations are diligently seeking ways to lower the injury rate for kids. Useful information is provided by the annual survey of high-school sports injuries done by the National Athletic Injury Reporting System (NAIRS) in conjunction with the National Trainers Association. However, even more accurate data are needed to identify specific injuries and their causes that make a sport unsafe.

Meanwhile, one of the major hopes of improving youth sports safety is the involvement of parents. In this book you will find many things you can do to make sports safer for your child and other children. All of these recommendations should be made part of your family sports safety program. Carrying out this program will take time and effort, but the result will be that sports are more fun for your kids and cause less anxiety for you.

◆   **YOUTH SPORTS PROGRAMS: ARE THEY DEDICATED TO SAFETY?**

Among school and nonschool sports programs, dedication to safety is a mixed bag. Many national organizations are undertaking safe-sport programs, of which Little League, Inc.'s program is an outstanding example. Started in 1990, this program offers each of the 160,000 teams in the United States a thirty-minute video on sports injuries, which is presented by a member of the American Orthopedic Society for Sports Medicine. An instructional booklet and follow-up examination for coaches are included. Other national youth sports organizations sponsor safety programs as well. The Amateur Hockey Association has made almost forty safety-related rule changes since 1983.

In addition, many local youth sports groups have educational programs that include safety. In my own state, the Youth Soccer League sponsors an excellent program that presents a workshop on preventing and treating injuries in youth soccer.

Still, many youth sports groups simply do not put enough emphasis on preventing injuries, especially when players under the age of thirteen are involved. It's true that these youngsters seldom suffer serious injuries, which occur more frequently in high-school sports. But it is imperative to instill safety measures and provide prevention programs early, when youngsters are just learning a sport. Their safety skills will become ingrained and serve them well in their teens. A positive example was set by the "pee wee" hockey leagues, which required youngsters to wear helmets and masks. These young athletes grew up with this protective equipment until wearing it became second nature.

In most sports, coaches are the key to injury prevention. However, we can't assume that today's coaches know all the answers to preventing injuries or even that they are actively pursuing that goal. The top priority of some coaches is to win at all costs—and the costs can be unnecessary, serious injuries. That's why it is most important for parents to meet with their youngster's coach and stress the need for injury prevention.

Obviously, youth sports organizations must intensify their efforts to improve safety. Parents can play a key role by encouraging these efforts from the youth sports groups with which their children are affiliated, whether in or out of school.

◆   **HOW SERIOUS ARE SPORTS INJURIES?**

There are two major types of physical injuries that occur in sports: the *acute* injury and the *overuse* injury. An acute injury is usually caused by abrupt force, such as impact with another athlete; a blow from a ball, puck, or stick; or a sudden twist that may sprain an ankle or tear a knee ligament. An overuse injury is a progressive condition caused by repetitive stress on one part of the body. An example is tendinitis in a baseball pitcher's elbow. Contact/collision sports like football have a high percentage of acute injuries, while noncontact sports like track are subject mostly to overuse injuries.

Generally, most acute sports injuries are minor bumps and bruises that heal quickly and don't require time off from the sport. But certain types of injuries require a young athlete to interrupt competition until recovery, particularly ankle sprains and injuries to the shoulder or knee. Of these, knee injuries cause the most long-term residual problems.

Overuse injuries, though unlikely to be permanent or require extensive treatment, may take many months to heal before a young athlete can return to competition.

Although the severity of injuries is related to the amount of force involved in a sport, it would be a mistake to assume that risks of serious injury are confined to contact/collision sports. It's true that football has the highest percentage of serious injuries. Wrestling and ice hockey are other high-risk sports. But many limited-impact sports, such as gymnastics, also have a significant percentage of severe injuries. There is a potential for serious injury in almost all types of sports, even those that are relatively safe. For example, overuse injuries are a major problem in track and cross-country running.

Another factor in the severity of sports injuries is the age of the young athlete. Kids who participate in youth-league sports, such as Little League baseball, range in age from four to thirteen. They rarely suffer serious injuries, which become more frequent when these youngsters get into high-school and college sports.

Always keep in mind that a physical sports injury usually carries with it an emotional injury as well. A blow to the youngster's confidence and self-esteem can't be measured by X rays and clinical examinations, but it can be even more serious than the physical injury itself. When a youngster is injured, parents should be aware of the possible emotional damage, because it is often kept hidden. You'll find recommendations for handling this problem in Chapter 11: *Guiding Your Youngster Through the "Injury Interaction."*

◆ YOUR GUIDE TO SPECIFIC SPORTS AND THEIR RISKS

Each sport has its own level of injury risk, and participants are susceptible to different types of injuries. One of the first steps parents can take to minimize sports injuries is to learn about the sport or sports in which their children want to participate. By knowing the sport's risks of injury and the specific injuries likely to occur, you can do a lot to minimize or prevent these injuries.

In addition to reading the following guide, you can gain first-hand knowledge of injury risks by attending several games of the sport in which your youngster is interested.

This guide has been adapted from the classification of sports developed by the American Academy of Pediatrics. There are three main categories:

1. Contact/Collision Sports
2. Limited Contact/Impact Sports
3. Noncontact Sports
   a) Strenuous
   b) Moderately Strenuous
   c) Nonstrenuous

For a complete list of the sports in each category see the box on page 10.

Comprehensive general guidelines for preventing injuries in these sports are provided in Chapter 7: *Nine Keys to Preventing Sports Injuries.* However, some sport-specific prevention tips are given in the following rundown:

◆ Contact/Collision Sports

These are sports that not only permit but actually require forceful physical contact. They are high-risk sports and injuries are inevitable. Players in these sports don't intentionally try to injure their opponents. But in football, for example, their primary goal is to hit opposing players so hard they can't perform their assignments. Some of the resulting injuries will be serious—and a few will cause permanent damage that can alter a young athlete's life.

SOCCER

Soccer is the most widely played international sport and one of the fastest growing sports in the United States. There are five million youngsters under nineteen playing soccer today.

Soccer is a high-speed endurance sport that is relatively safe, with an injury rate about half that of football. However, high schools have a higher injury rate than youth leagues because of the more physical play.

Very few soccer injuries are serious. However, even though soccer rules forbid forceful contact with another player, collisions are frequent. According to the *American Journal of Sports Medicine*[1] rule violations cause 30 percent of soccer injuries, while poor field conditions cause another 25 percent.

The most frequent injuries in soccer are:

Lower-Extremity Injuries (68%). Of these, ankle sprains account for the most time lost in soccer. Another common injury is the "soccer foot" or "soccer toe," caused by overuse. This is not a permanent injury. Knee-ligament tears are the most serious lower-extremity injury in high-school soccer, but they do not occur frequently to pre-high-school players because their bodies are more elastic.

Upper-Extremity Injuries (15%). Shoulder bruises and

[1]Keller, Cary S., M.D., Frank R. Noyes, M.D., and C. Ralph Buncher, ScD. "The Medical Aspects of Soccer Injury Epidemiology." *American Journal of Sports Medicine,* Vol. 16, Supplement 1, 1988: pp. S-105 to S-112.

How Sports are Classified

1. CONTACT/COLLISION SPORTS

Soccer	*Boys' Lacrosse*
Wrestling	*Field Hockey*
Ice Hockey	*Martial Arts*
Football	*Boxing*
Rugby	*Rodeo*

2. LIMITED CONTACT/IMPACT SPORTS

Basketball	*Volleyball*
Baseball	*Bicycling*
Softball	*Diving*
Gymnastics	*Field Events*
Downhill Skiing	*Figure Skating*
Cross-Country Skiing	*Roller Skating*
Water Skiing	*Squash*
Equestrian Sports	*Racquetball*
Girls' Lacrosse	*Cheerleading*

3. NONCONTACT SPORTS

Strenuous

Running	*Shot Put*
Swimming	*Discus*
Rowing	*Javelin*
Tennis	*Dancing*
Weight Lifting	

Moderately Strenuous

Badminton	*Table Tennis*
Curling	*Hiking*

Nonstrenuous

Golf	*Riflery*
Archery	

sprains are common, but there are few separations or dislocations. Fractured wrists can also occur.

Head Injuries (10%). These are seldom anything more than mild concussions.

Trunk Injuries (7%). Mostly bumps and bruises.

Prevention: Conditioning, good officiating, shin guards, and proper shoes.

WRESTLING

Wrestling is one of the great sports of ancient times that continues to grow in popularity today. An estimated 250,000 U.S. youngsters compete in high-school wrestling.

Although wrestling has many benefits for the young athlete, it also has a high injury rate at the high-school level. (In youth-league wrestling injuries are minimal.) In 1983, J. Estwanik, a prominent sports physician, reported a 23-percent injury rate among North Carolina high-school wrestlers. Only 6.3 percent of these injuries were major.

Wrestling injuries to be aware of are:

Knee Injuries. The most common wrestling injury, and it can be serious.

Hand and Finger Injuries. Very common.

Head and Face Injuries. "Cauliflower ear" is a typical wrestling injury, but it can be eliminated almost completely by wearing headgear in practice and competition.

Bloody Noses. Common but of no consequence.

Neck Injuries. Simple sprains are common, but serious neck injuries are rare.

Shoulder Injuries. A common injury ranging from a strain to dislocation.

Weight Loss. Last-minute, excessive weight reduction to qualify for lower weight classes is one of the most critical problems in youth wrestling. It is covered fully in Chapter 6: *Five Special Medical Considerations.*

Prevention: Because of the power, force, and torque placed on the body in wrestling, injuries cannot be avoided. But in addition to following general safety procedures, wrestlers can reduce their injuries by doing supervised strength training and wearing protective headgear.

ICE HOCKEY

There are 300,000 hockey players and 12,000 teams in the United States. In Canada, there are more than a million players. Hockey is a high-speed sport, and the confines of the rink require skillful performance to avoid injury.

As with football, there are few major calamities in ice hockey played by younger children in the youth leagues. The troublesome injuries begin with the teenage years. Although tragic injuries were reduced when protective headgear was made mandatory, another problem was created. Players developed a false sense of security from their helmets and face masks. They began to hit the boards and each other with less caution. This recklessness has produced a shocking increase in head and neck injuries—including broken necks.

There are six frequent types of ice hockey injuries:

Head Injuries. Despite the higher rate of head injuries, the use of helmets prevents most of them from being serious.

Neck Injuries. The young neck is not protected by a helmet and is not strong enough to protect itself as readily as in more mature years. This makes it more vulnerable to serious injury, especially when a youngster plays recklessly under the illusion that the helmet will prevent any injury.

Hockey goalies face a serious risk: The puck can strike them in the throat. Even though they are protected by neck guards—which are mandatory in both youth-league and high-school hockey—physicians, trainers, and emergency medical technicians (EMTs) should be prepared for this emergency.

Facial Injuries. The face mask has reduced these injuries but not completely eliminated them.

Shoulder Injuries. The shoulder is at high risk in boys' ice hockey. Separated shoulders are common and dislocations sometimes occur.

Elbow Injuries. Traumatic bursitis (inflammation of the soft, fluid-filled sac that minimizes friction near joints) is common, and there is an occasional fracture.

Wrist Injuries. Wrist fractures occur frequently, and are critical when the *navicular* bone is fractured.

Groin and Thigh Injuries. Hockey players are very susceptible to these injuries.

Knee Injuries. Not as common as in football, but they are still frequent. Generally, the injury is less devastating and limited to the ligaments that heal more readily.

Ankle Injuries. Fairly common, but they almost always mend well with no permanent problem.

Prevention: A prime cause of hockey injuries is uncontrolled violence. Prevention begins with coaches and game officials who insist on strict adherence to safe rules of play.

FOOTBALL

Serious injuries begin with high-school football. Players under the age of fourteen seldom suffer anything more than bumps, bruises, and sprains. In fact, in the Pop Warner leagues for these youngsters, football is actually as safe as any other sport in this age bracket. In thirty years of caring for football players under the age of fourteen, I have treated only two major injuries: a leg fracture and a freak knee injury. Both injuries healed without permanent damage.

At these ages, young bodies are so rubbery and elastic that they more often stretch than tear and lack sufficient weight or power to injure another player. Just as important, these youngsters haven't yet developed the aggressive instincts that can lead to injuries.

This doesn't mean that parents should be unconcerned and uninvolved if their under-age-fourteen child is playing football. For example, injuries are likely when oversized or over-mature youngsters are permitted to play on a team, especially if some of the other kids are undersized. Teams should be balanced physically rather than only by chronological age.

High-school football is a totally different story. It has the highest injury rate of all sports, including other contact-collision sports. Every team is likely to have some major injuries. All of the players will suffer bruises and contusions, while one-third will have more serious injuries. This adds up to a lot of injury and pain when you consider that over 1.3 million youngsters play high-school football in the United States. The National Athletic Trainers Association reported in 1989 that there were approximately half a million high-school football injuries a year—and that one-third of these injuries sidelined the player for three weeks or more. Football deaths have averaged ten a year between 1970 and 1990—most of them occurring to high-school players.

How come? Football is a hard-hitting power sport where eleven players drive forward to force their opponents back or confine them. The amount of force involved and the angle and speed of the thrust create the high injury rate.

So why should you allow your kid to play football? As with any activity, you should weigh the rewards and values against the risks. Football has many rewards that make it worthwhile. They include personal satisfaction, self-esteem, personal inner strength, self-confidence, social prestige, and being part of a team. For those who *want* to play football there is nothing quite so satisfying as blocking an opponent so hard that he is taken out of the play or carrying the ball past a tackler who is trying to stop you. To be part of a team that drives over the goal against a powerful opponent leaves memories that are relived with warm satisfaction for years.

This doesn't mean that high-school football is right for every youngster. We'll discuss that important point in the next two chapters.

What are the most serious injuries in football? There are six that are most likely to have permanent consequences:

Head Injuries. Only boxers suffer more head injuries than football players. Most are mild concussions of little consequence. But some are serious and even fatal— each year there are several football deaths caused by head injuries.

Fortunately, rule changes in football have reduced the frequency of head injuries. One important change outlawed "spearing"—that is, using one's head as a weapon to tackle or block an opposing player. The number of deaths and amount of permanent damage can also be reduced by good coaching and early recognition of a head injury when it occurs. But because of football's inherent nature, such injuries can never be entirely eliminated.

Neck Injuries. Stretch injuries to the neck are frequent. Although most are not serious, some can have permanent consequences. The most catastrophic injury in football is the "broken neck," which can result in quadriplegia—paralysis from the neck down. Although the number of broken necks in football has been reduced by more than 100 percent in recent years—because of the rule changes mentioned earlier—there is still an average of ten quadriplegic accidents in football every year.

Shoulder Injuries. These injuries are among the most common in football. When they occur, their seriousness is often not recognized immediately.

Abdominal Injury. Although this injury is infrequent in football, the possibility of a ruptured spleen is always present. Immediate recognition of this injury is the key to preventing permanent effects.

Knee Injuries. These are the most frequent and disabling extremity injuries in football. One in four high-school football players will suffer some type of knee injury. According to a National Athletic Trainers Association study, about fifteen thousand high-school football knee injuries require surgery each year—almost 70 percent of *all* operations performed on high-school football players. (See Chapter 17 for more about knee injuries.)

Ankle Injuries. Much playing time is lost from these very common football injuries, a small percentage of which can trouble the athlete later on in life.

Prevention: Conditioning, including strength training, is the best way to prevent football injuries. Good technique, equipment, and playing conditions are also essential.

RUGBY

Although rugby is played in U.S. colleges, it is uncommon in high schools and youth leagues. Rugby players wear no protective equipment, but they still have a lower injury rate than football players. However, rugby does have a high risk of injuries to the head, the large joints, the shoulder, and the knee.

Prevention: As with football, conditioning, technique, equipment, and playing conditions are the most important preventive factors.

BOYS' LACROSSE

Lacrosse, a game that was originated by Native Americans before white settlers arrived, has become a popular sport in the United States. Injuries are similar to those in ice hockey and football, with about half of the players suffering at least one injury that requires medical attention. Shoulder injuries are the most frequent, and knee and ankle injuries are also a problem. Seventy percent of lacrosse injuries are minor, but the goalie is vulnerable to throat injuries from a direct hit with the ball.

Prevention: As well as conditioning, technique, and safe

equipment, adherence to the rules will help to prevent boys' lacrosse injuries.

FIELD HOCKEY

In the United States, field hockey is a female sport. The most common serious injuries are to the knee, back, and face. Knee injuries are likely to involve the *anterior cruciate ligament,* resulting in a major problem. Stick injuries to the face also can be serious, while less serious injuries occur to the shin, foot, and ankle.

Prevention: The best preventives are conditioning and stretching, adherence to the rules, and good equipment, including mouth guards and shin pads.

MARTIAL ARTS

Although far more popular in the Orient where they originated, martial arts—such as karate, kung-fu, judo, and tae kwon do—are practiced by about 200,000 Americans. For children, the injury rate is under 1 percent—much lower than that for adults. The most frequent injuries are to the shoulder, elbow, and wrist. Broken toes are also common.

Prevention: It's important to supervise the combatants to make sure they don't use maneuvers that are beyond their experience and training. Padded mats are also important.

BOXING

Boxing is the only sport where the primary goal is to injure your opponent. Despite this, boxing has a 50-percent injury rate, which is lower than that of some other contact/collision sports. As with most sports, youngsters from ten to thirteen years of age suffer very few injuries from boxing. But if they continue boxing, permanent brain damage can occur that may not show itself for years. To be sure, boxing can be made safer with mouth guards; headgear; and heavier, thumbless gloves, as well as point systems and restrictions on head punches. But in my opinion, the potential for permanent damage still outweighs the positive aspects of the sport.

RODEO

Although there are no statistics on injuries to young rodeo riders, it must be considered one of the high-risk sports.

◆ Limited Contact/Impact Sports

This class includes team and individual sports that require strength and permit body contact on a limited basis. But even though contact is limited, *all sports in this category have a high percentage of injuries*. Serious injuries can occur that can change the life of the injured youngster.

BASKETBALL

More than twenty-two million Americans play basketball, making it one of the most popular team sports in the United States. This is a high-speed endurance sport requiring an extraordinary combination of balance, agility, and strength. Although theoretically a noncontact sport, basketball has become much more of a contact sport in recent years. Reports indicate that up to two-thirds of basketball participants will sustain at least one injury, but 90 percent of these injuries are minor and do not result from contact with other players. According to the National Athletic Trainers Association, only 2 percent of total injuries required surgery.

The most common injuries in basketball occur to the lower extremities.

Ankle Injuries. Ligament sprains of the ankle are the most frequent basketball injury, but with good care they heal well.

Foot Injuries. Blisters, abrasions, and skin conditions of the foot are common but insignificant. Stress fractures of the navicular bone and the base of the fifth metatarsal (see Illustrations 31 and 32 on pages 293–294) are more serious.

Knee Injuries. These injuries are second in frequency to ankle injuries and the most serious injuries in basketball, resulting in the highest number of missed games. "Jumper's Knee" is one of the less serious knee injuries but probably the most common. Tall, athletic female teenagers are more susceptible than male players to very disabling knee injuries that require major ligament surgery.

Back Injuries. Mostly back sprains, these injuries can create major problems.

Shoulder Injuries. These occur mostly from falls and are seldom serious.

Finger Injuries. These are quite common and require an accurate diagnosis and good care.

Eye Injuries. Fairly frequent because of contact with fingers, finger nails, elbows, and heads.

Prevention: Basketball injuries are difficult to prevent, but endurance training, adequate pregame warm-ups, and stretching can help to reduce overuse injuries, while good officiating can keep contact injuries down.

BASEBALL

Four-and-a-half million amateurs participate in the great American pastime, half of them under the age of thirteen. Baseball is a relatively safe sport, with a lower injury rate than most major sports. The most common injury risk is to the young pitcher, who can develop "Little League elbow" or a painful shoulder from throwing curve balls or throwing other types of pitches to excess. In spite of plenty of publicity and warnings about this problem, it continues to persist.

The most serious injuries in baseball are to the chest and head, from being hit by a pitched or batted ball. Some of these injuries are fatal, and the number of deaths among young baseball players is second only to those in football. For the most part, however, baseball injuries consist of bumps, bruises, and fractures.

Prevention: The protective helmet worn by batters helps to prevent the most serious injuries to the head, and further protection can be provided by face masks and a softer baseball (see page 130). Breakaway bases also help to prevent injuries. Young pitchers can protect themselves by avoiding overuse of their arms.

SOFTBALL

The two most common serious injuries in softball are ankle and finger fractures. Severe injuries from being hit by the softer ball are less common.

Prevention: See Baseball above.

GYMNASTICS

The injury risk for young gymnasts is one of the highest in sports. Despite this, gymnastics was one of the fastest growing sports of the 1980s, and about 500,000 youngsters participate in local, regional, and national competition. They usually start between the ages of five and eight and may continue into their twenties.

Parents of youngsters interested in this sport should be aware of the potential problems. Acute traumatic injuries can occur from falls and dismounts. Overuse injuries can occur from highly intense year-round training. Besides the everyday bumps, bruises, and strains, there can be serious fractures, dislocations, and back problems such as *spondylolisthesis.* Torn ligaments are not unusual. Although some catastrophic injuries to the head and neck occur, their frequency has been sharply reduced since the use of the trampoline was discontinued in gymnastics. These are dangerous devices and should never be used by young gymnasts.

Overuse injuries are common in gymnastics, including *osteochondritis* of the elbow or knee, *epiphysitis* of the spine and knee, and stress fractures. These injuries are described in Part IV: *Home Reference Guide to Sports Injuries—From Head to Toe.* Severe dieting and weight loss are also hazardous for young gymnasts.

Prevention: Important preventive factors are secure

equipment, skilled spotters, thorough stretching, strength training, and staying within one's capabilities.

DOWNHILL SKIING

About ten million people in the United States participate in recreational downhill skiing. Every year, more than 500,000 injuries are reported, with almost half of them occurring to children. Most of these injuries are caused by falls, only about 15 percent by collisions.

The most serious skiing injuries are to the knee ligaments, and their frequency is increasing. Children also suffer quite a few fractures in skiing, but these injuries seldom leave the residual disability that can result from knee ligament damage.

A common skiing injury is "skier's thumb," an injury to the inside ligament of the thumb caused by the thumb being caught in the ski-pole strap during a spill.

In competitive skiing, shoulder dislocations are frequent, and some head injuries have been reported. *Prevention:* Good instruction is important, because the more skilled the skier the less likelihood of an accident. Youngsters must learn to ski "in control" on appropriate slopes and to obey warnings from the ski patrol. Good, well-fitted equipment and clothing are also essential. Youngsters should not be allowed to ski when they are fatigued.

CROSS-COUNTRY SKIING

This form of skiing is an increasingly popular sport with a very low injury rate among youngsters.

WATER SKIING

Water skiing is more hazardous to the recreational skier than to the competitive skier. Knee ligament injuries are frequent and can cause long-term problems. Major muscle tears in the groin and thigh also occur, while female skiers sometimes suffer traumatic water douches (see page 263). Propeller injuries and drowning are quite rare.

Prevention: Life jackets, adequate boat speed, and an untangled line are important injury preventives. There should be standard signals for communication between the skier and the observer in the boat, and skiers should only do maneuvers that are within their ability.

EQUESTRIAN SPORTS

Parents should be aware that both competitive and recreational equestrian sports have a high injury risk; in fact, they are ranked among the most dangerous sports along with motorcycle and automobile racing. Despite this, equestrian sports are popular—more than eight million people in the United States mount a horse at least once a year.

The most severe injuries are to the head and spine. Severe upper-extremity fractures also occur. Injuries to the major joints occur most frequently when jumping is involved. In jumping, there is also the risk that the horse can crush or trample the rider.

Inexperienced children and teenagers have the most equestrian accidents, including being kicked, thrown from the horse, and dragged by the horse while the foot is caught in a stirrup.

Prevention: Hard hats, supervised training, and proper matching of horse and rider are essential. So is maintenance of equipment.

GIRLS' LACROSSE

Like boys' lacrosse, the girls' version uses sticks and a hard ball thrown at high speed. However, girls' lacrosse has a much lower injury rate because of its no-contact rule. Facial fractures are the most serious injury but occur infrequently. More common are usually insignificant hand injuries and sprained ankles. As with all running and pivot sports, there can be knee ligament and cartilage injuries, but they are far less frequent than in field hockey.

Prevention: As with boys' lacrosse, girls' lacrosse injuries can be prevented through conditioning, good technique, safe equipment, and adherence to the rules.

VOLLEYBALL

This is a high-speed sport with explosive action requiring contorted movements and dangerous jumping and lunging. Injuries can be caused by player collisions, floor burns, and hard-driven balls. Every part of the body is vulnerable to injury, particularly fingers, ankles, knees, and shoulders. Overuse injuries include "jumper's knee" and shin splints.

Prevention: In addition to conditioning and use of knee pads, coordinated play is all-important in preventing volleyball injuries.

BICYCLING

Cycling is a rapidly growing competitive sport divided into three categories: track racing, tour racing, and all-terrain racing. Head injuries from falls are the most serious injuries in this sport, but they can be reduced by the use of helmets. Overuse injuries can occur to the knees, arms, and groin.

Prevention: In addition to helmets, important factors are a proper fit between bicycle and rider, bicycle maintenance, conditioning, avoiding fatigue, proper clothing, and alertness to possible collisions.

DIVING

This sport, which requires form, rhythm, and grace, is subject to very few injuries. However, there are hazards to watch out for: hitting the board, spraining the back, overstretching the muscles, and diving in shallow water (which occurs, sometimes tragically, in recreational diving).

Prevention: Conditioning, strength training, and skill in performance.

FIELD EVENTS

In the *high jump*, back injuries, muscle pulls, and "jumper's knee" are all common complaints. But, for the most part, this sport is quite safe.

Though not injury free, the *pole vault* is also a safe sport if properly coached. Correct positioning of the bar, a secure vaulting box, and a well-placed, padded landing surface are essential. Although most injuries occur on landing, muscles can be pulled during takeoff, and a broken pole can cause injury as well.

In the *long jump* and *triple jump*, landing injuries are most common, including ankle and knee sprains, back sprains, and occasional fractures. The effort of the jump itself can cause pulls and tears of muscles and tendons.

Prevention: Conditioning, strength training, good technique, and a clear field area will all help to reduce injuries.

FIGURE SKATING

Figure skating has been increasingly popular in the United States ever since Dr. Tenley Albright brought home the first U.S. Olympic gold medal in the sport in 1956. Overuse injuries are far more common than acute injuries; constant repetitions of specific moves and jumps can cause stress injuries ranging from simple strains to stress fractures.

Prevention: Conditioning, proper coaching, and progressive skills training are key preventives. Older skaters should work on strength training.

ROLLER SKATING

This is a growing competitive sport among youngsters. With the increase in individual and couples competition, skateboard competition, and the use of in-line rollerblades has come an increase in injuries. The most serious of these are fractures. A 1983 study estimated the cost of roller-skating injuries to be more than one-hundred million dollars annually.

Prevention: Wearing elbow and knee pads and using caution in the learning stages of skating.

SQUASH/RACQUETBALL

The major danger in these sports is an eye injury, but this risk has lessened since 1987, when players were required to wear protective glasses. Other injuries are ankle sprains, knee injuries, and tendinitis of the wrist. *Prevention:* Eye goggles are a must.

CHEERLEADING

Although not officially classified as a sport, cheerleading meets all the criteria for athletic activity. There are more than 600,000 cheerleaders in the United States, with about 150,000 attending high-school summer camps every year. In some areas of the country, cheerleaders begin at the age of eight. According to the 1990 edition of *Consumer Product Safety Commission Report,* a government publication, cheerleaders suffered sixty-seven hundred injuries in 1985, most commonly to the ankle and lower back. Catastrophic injuries to the neck and back from serious falls have also been reported.
Prevention: Conditioning, safety rules, and good coaching are key factors in prevention. Pyramid and tumbling stunts should not be performed without thorough training.

◆   Noncontact Sports

Most injuries in noncontact sports are caused by overuse rather than impact. However, there are a small percentage of impact injuries, such as falling on hurdles, hitting one's head on a diving board, or dropping a weight on one's foot.

Noncontact sports come in three varieties: strenuous, moderately strenuous, and nonstrenuous.

Strenuous Noncontact Sports

These are sports that keep physicians very busy. Most of them are individual sports in which young athletes must perform at the peak of their mental and physical ability, and injuries occur regularly because of the personal push to excel and the limitations of young bodies. "Do your best" is still good advice, but youngsters must also be educated in the best control and care of their bodies.

RUNNING

Children are now starting in distance running as young as ten, often under parental pressure. This is risky. Although complaints about normal aches are minor, you should be alert to such dangers as heat exhaustion and dehydration. Teenage runners suffer the usual overuse injuries of the sport. Forty-two percent of the complaints concern the knee; 28 percent, the leg (such as shin splints and stress fractures); and 20 percent, the foot. Most of these injuries belong in the nuisance category—they are frustrating but not disabling.
Prevention: Special care by parents and coaches to avoid extended training.

SWIMMING

Swimming is the most popular recreational sport in the United States, with an estimated 120 million participants. Competitive swimming is also a growing sport, and the sports medical world is increasingly concerned about the high incidence of injuries. Many of these injuries are overuse problems caused by the intensive training that young swimmers must go through. Training sometimes begins in infancy and competitive swimming starts at age eight. A training schedule for the average youngster will include swimming up to five thousand yards during each session.

The most frequent injury is "swimmer's shoulder," a form of tendinitis. "Swimmer's ear" is also common, as is "breast-stroke knee," a strain on the inner side of the knee.

Prevention: Progressive conditioning is essential; excessive training should be avoided.

ROWING

The most frequent complaints are back strain and knee strain.

Prevention: Conditioning, stretching, and strength training.

TENNIS

There is very little risk to the average young tennis player beyond the usual aches, pains, and sprains. However, when players reach regional and national competition, injury problems become more intense. Most frequently affected are the foot, knee, hand, and shoulder.

Prevention: Conditioning and overuse avoidance.

WEIGHT LIFTING

With youngsters, weight lifting is part of strength training rather than a competitive sport. Weight training injuries are discussed in Chapter 6.

SHOT PUT/DISCUS/JAVELIN

These three field events are subject to the same types of injuries because they all involve throwing. Hand injuries include blisters, joint sprains, and tendinitis. Tendinitis of the shoulder and sprains of the trunk and back can also occur. Lower-extremity injuries are not common.

Prevention: Strength training, good technique, and avoidance of excessive practice are the keys to preventing injuries in these sports.

DANCING/BALLET[2]

It's a fact that there are more young dance students in the United States than there are young football players. This athletic activity starts as early as five or six, requiring a discipline that becomes more intense and severe as the student progresses. Dancing calls for enormous dedication and personal sacrifice.

The injury risk is not great in younger children; the more significant injuries occur in adolescence. These are overuse injuries such as back strain, hip tendinitis, thigh strain and tendinitis, muscular strain, knee sprain and tendinitis, and kneecap stress. Other common injuries are stress fractures in the area of the tibia, ankle sprains, foot sprains, and inflammation of the first metatarsal joint. However, these are minor injuries that don't last long. There can be acute injuries from falling and infrequent major injuries to the knee and ankle.

Prevention: Conditioning and stretching. Youngsters who lift other dancers should also do strength training.

Moderately Strenuous Noncontact Sports

Of the four sports in this category—badminton, curling, table tennis, and hiking—only hiking presents significant injury risk: the danger of frostbite or hypothermia in freezing weather (see page 138 for more information).

Nonstrenuous Noncontact Sports

Very few injuries occur to youngsters in these sports—golf, archery, and riflery. However, back disorders can be a problem in golf, and there are some overuse injuries to the hand and shoulder in riflery and archery.

---

[2]Dance is considered a sport by most sports medical experts and by the American Pediatric Assocation. It is a very physical art with a high rate of injuries.

2

Introducing Your Child to Sports

◆

Y our *Michael* is four years old. He's not into competitive sports at this tender age. But both boys and girls *are* getting involved in sports at earlier and earlier ages. So before you know it, you may be asking yourself:

- Should Michael participate in competitive sports at all?
- If so, what sports would suit him best?
- At what age should he start them?
- What should be my role as a parent?

Here's help with these important questions.

◆ SHOULD YOUR CHILD COMPETE IN SPORTS?

Ultimately, of course, only you can answer that question. You know your child better than anyone else. But there are some guidelines and considerations that can help you make the right decision without relying too much on what you would like to see your child doing.

A large majority of children and youths today want to participate in sports of some kind. Some are eager for team sports, while others enjoy individual competition. Still other children are not physically competitive and have little interest in sports. For the most part, they have no problem avoiding the athletic field; but, unfortunately, some are pressed into competitive sports by parents trying to fulfill their own dreams of grandeur.

◆ The Value of Sports

For many children, sports competition is a natural part of their development. Being on a team or involved in an individual sport is a growth experience. Belonging is a vital need in life, a need that sports participation can help to satisfy.

Young people learn the reality of life on the playing field. Sports can build self-confidence and help to give your child the self-esteem that is so essential for healthy development and personal survival. There is definitely a sense of pride that develops from being on a team or performing well in an individual sport. Properly handled by you and your children's coach, this pride will provide an identity that can add immeasurably to future success.

Every sport has its own special rewards. To many youngsters, the individual discipline of hours of swimming or miles of road-running can bring about personal triumphs of unmeasured value in future years. In team sports, throwing a successful block in football or checking an opponent hard on the boards in ice hockey brings a feeling of accomplishment that every parent should try to understand.

The Distortion of Sports Values

Some child psychiatrists and psychologists believe that children should not participate in organized sports at all. In their opinion, imagination and development are better stimulated by free and unorganized play.

I disagree with that position. The concept of organized sports for children is sound. But there are serious problems associated with competitive sports for young people today, and parents should be aware of them. Among them are:

- Failing to give top priority to safety in youth sports.
- Exploiting children to further the goals of adults.
- Coaching by untrained, unsuitable people.
- Emphasizing "win at all costs" rather than the value of participation.
- Starting children too early in a sport, before they are old enough to grasp the concepts.
- Failing to perceive kids' desires and pushing them into sports which they eventually grow to hate.
- Permitting youngsters to overtrain—the "overuse syndrome"—which leads to injuries.
- Failing to recognize the loss of self-esteem and self-confidence which can come from making an embarrassing mistake (like kicking a soccer ball and missing completely) and being derided by spectators, coaches, parents, etc.
- Glorifying young sports competitors at the expense of youngsters accomplished in other areas.
- Growing commercialization of high-school sports, including college-type recruiting and corporate sponsorship for live national broadcasts of big games. (Many of the problems afflicting college sports are now showing up in high-school sports.)

All of these problems should send a vital message to you as a parent: *Give your kids thorough guidance to help them establish sound sports values.* This is especially important when you see that your child has a strong competitive spirit at an early age. The minds of competitive children are filled with endless fantasies of their amazing exploits at the Olympics, the World Series, Wimbledon, or the Super Bowl. These kids are exploding with energy— energy that needs to be harnessed and properly directed into healthy channels by both parent and coach. This guidance can propel them into personal accomplishments and security without undue damage to their bodies *or* their minds.

◆ How to Know if Your Child Wants to Compete

Your child should only compete if he or she wants to compete. As parents, you must keep an open mind on the subject. If you have already decided for your child, you will tend to disregard signals indicating that you may have made the wrong decision. Be willing to check what you want and listen to your child.

Looking for Signals

Usually it's not difficult to determine if your children want to participate in competitive sports. But you may not get an early answer. In that case, don't force the issue, but continue to support their interests and wait for them to give you signals or tell you directly what their feelings are about sports. Chances are that a child who is constantly throwing a ball or roughhousing with friends will be a natural sports competitor. Another sign is whether the child enjoys watching sports events on television. Children who seem far more interested in reading, playing a musical instrument, or other nonathletic pursuits may not want to get into sports.

Once children are already involved in a sport, it's fairly easy to determine if they're happy or not. Some positive clues to look for:

- They're eager to tell you what happened in practice or a game.
- They take their baseball glove or tennis racket to bed.
- They practice at home.

On the other hand, alarm bells should go off if:

- They practically have to be dragged to practice.
- There's no response when you ask if the practice or the game went well.
- They take poor care of their equipment.

Naturally, you should be concerned with any childhood signs that something is not right. Sports may not be the problem, but investigate that possibility.

When your child does show an interest in a specific sport, and you believe it is appropriate, your support and encouragement are essential. How many times do we see junior-high and high-school competitions with only a handful of parents watching and cheering? Be there if you can. Remember, these childhood years go by very quickly.

Of course, some kids are exceptions—they don't want their parents around during a game. I recall a young lacrosse player who went to pieces when her mother arrived for a game and a young wrestler who actually vomited every time his parents came to a match. So don't make assumptions—be sure your child wants you there before you show up.

Exposing Your Kids to Sports

If your kids are interested in sports but have not yet developed preferences for specific sports, give them time and expose them to as many different sports as you can. Get them a baseball bat, a football, a soccer ball. Take them to tennis matches, horse shows, swim meets. They will eventually find the sport in which they want to participate. Or they may end up deciding they prefer to watch rather than participate. If so, don't push them.

Watching television is another way in which children will often develop their sports interests, since in many homes entire weekends are centered around televised sports events. Keep in mind, though, that some types of sports are rarely televised, so children must be exposed to them in other ways.

◆ WHAT SPORTS FOR YOUR CHILD?

The dreams going through a parent's head when a child is born frequently set the stage for sports activities in the future. Fathers especially are prone to think about sports for their newborn, and have been known to bring footballs or tennis rackets to the hospital! They are projecting their own sports fantasies onto their child, which may be very unwise.

Parents should wait until their child develops some

individuality before even thinking about sports. You may notice that at the age of two or three your child loves to dance around the kitchen, may try to hit a ball with a plastic bat, or wants to play catch. But for the most part kids' actions at these ages are simply a generalized expression of physical activity, without any focus on a specific sport. If you encourage their activity, their response to certain sports may give you clues to what they like or dislike.

◆   Choosing the Right Sport

In considering specific sports, make sure you choose a sport in which your youngster is ready to participate. Forcing your very young into a particular sport—whether directly or indirectly—can start early conflicts within the child. These conflicts may not surface for years, but they may cause psychological damage.

So keep your antenna up. Try to read your child, listen to your spouse, and don't assume that your sports interests are the same as those of your child. If you're a single parent, talk to other parents and to your child's friends.

It's a good idea to encourage children to try several sports in the early years. Each sport has unique skills. Exposure to these different skills can make it easier for you to recognize which sports they enjoy and perform well.

Consciously or not, parents often lead their children toward the sports they played when young or enjoy now. There's nothing wrong with that. In fact, if you all play tennis, ski, or skate, your youngster is likely to join the fun. But be careful not to push a *reluctant* youngster into a sport simply because it is "your" sport—boredom and resentment may be the result. Remember that your child is an individual, not an extension of yourself.

Look for these clues to indicate what sports he or she might be interested in:

- A youngster who loves to tumble, wrestle, and roughhouse may find contact/collision sports the most satisfying.
- A child who steps away from this kind of physical contact

may find more rewards in gentler sports that emphasize skill over strength.

• Some youths are happy diving off the board, hitting tennis balls against the wall, or running on the road. They're more likely to be interested in individual sports than in team sports.

Female Sport Choices

Before you go into shock over some of your daughter's unconventional sports choices, recognize that more and more girls are becoming active in power sports like soccer, basketball, softball, field hockey, and ice hockey. There's a strong trend toward more team competition among girls, and colleges are offering more athletic scholarships to women every year. (Special medical considerations for young female athletes are discussed in Chapter 6.)

Sports Cost Money

Almost any sport your children get into will require money. But some sports are more costly than others. For individual sports in particular, you may have to lay out hundreds of dollars for lessons, practice sessions, and equipment. For team sports you must come up with money for uniforms and equipment and possibly travel. So be sure to check into the costs of any sports you and your youngster may be considering. Once you know these costs, you can measure them against such factors as your budget, your child's desire to pursue this particular sport, and your own willingness to pay the cost.

Medical insurance is another financial factor to consider. Family insurance is usually the primary coverage in individual, youth-league, and school sports. However, youth leagues may offer reasonably priced insurance for participating youngsters, and schools may have an insurance program that provides back-up medical coverage for injured athletes.

With today's high health-care costs, be sure you understand what insurance coverage is available for your youngster's sports injuries. If you have no health insurance, discuss the problem with the school athletic director or the youth-league director. You don't want to end up with a financial crisis over a broken wrist or sprained ankle.

Making It a Family Affair

As much as possible, choosing sports for your children should be a coordinated process. Hold family meetings to discuss the pros and cons of different sports. Express any personal concerns you may have about particular sports. These might include:

- The extent to which your youngster is interested in the sport
- The time involved—both yours and the child's
- The financial cost
- The availability of the sport in your community

◆ Dealing with the Permission Problem

As your children grow older, they often get involved in specific sports on their own, without your input. Usually it happens at school: Your ten-year-old *John* is in a group that plays baseball and he joins the activity. You may never openly give your consent and John may not ask for it. As a result, he doesn't know how you feel about it and may end up plagued by insecurity and doubt.

So if you allow your youngster to compete in a sport, give your permission explicitly and positively. Your child needs your approval and support for every sport in which he or she participates, whether youth-league sports, school sports, or individual sports. This is a crucial time for you to encourage your young athlete. Your support provides a feeling of security that allows the youngster to focus on good execution of skills, which can minimize danger of injury.

When You Feel Like Saying No

If you're happy about your child's choice of sport, you'll have no problem giving your enthusiastic permission. But what if you're *not* happy about it—what if you object for some reason to the sport in which your child wants to participate? That's more troublesome.

Let's narrow it down: A principal reason parents object to their child's choice of a sport is their fear of injury. This fear arises most often with sports that have high injury rates: football, ice hockey, wrestling, and other contact/collision sports.

What should you do in this situation? After all, you are responsible for your child's well-being and you are in charge. Whatever you do should create a secure, positive experience for your youngster rather than a negative, threatening one.

So should you allow your child to play in a sport with a high injury rate? You must deal with this question yourself, because a youngster who is enthusiastic about a sport is unlikely to be too concerned about its dangers. You are the one who must understand the injury risks of specific sports, as discussed in Chapter 1.

I believe that in spite of the risks, youngsters should be allowed to play and even be encouraged to play in contact/collision sports *if they meet two important criteria*: One, they are strongly motivated to participate in this sport; two, they are "physical"—that is, they enjoy forceful contact and rough-and-tumble play.

Most people who have participated in contact/collision sports during their youth will tell you it was worth it. As was pointed out earlier, these sports can be valuable in maturing young people and helping them adjust to the real world. True, these sports are sometimes injurious. But so is life itself.

◆ WHAT'S THE BEST AGE TO START EACH SPORT?

As was said earlier, unless there is obviously a specific direction in which a child wants to go (such as figure skating), it's best for young children to get involved in several different sports at an early age because they're more likely to end up with a sport they really enjoy. Even those sports they drop will leave them with valuable skills.

Although there are no data for determining precisely when a child should start a specific sport, the following guidelines are based on the extensive experience and observation of sports medical professionals.

THREE TO FOUR

Dance, figure skating, and swimming are examples of sports that often start as early as age three. It is particularly important at this age for sports to be a fun experience, so there should be plenty of playtime along with the training. Youngsters who persevere through these early years often continue to a successful career. In my experience, however, there is a high dropout rate. Parents should be alert for signs that the child wants out—sometimes it doesn't become obvious for many years.

FIVE TO SIX

These are fledgling years for such sports as skiing, soccer, gymnastics, judo, hockey, and figure skating—and they are great years for family participation. When the program is kept at a truly recreational level, most youngsters at these ages will participate happily. Developing skills and fulfilling the need for belonging are keys to these early programs.

SEVEN TO EIGHT

These are years when natural instincts for athletics begin to show themselves. It's a good time to introduce team sports. With most youngsters, it's too early to expect skills like baseball pitching, but not too early for skills in sports that involve kicking, such as soccer. Youngsters who begin team sports this early are often more mature and developed than those who have started these sports at later ages. But this is no reason to push your kids into team sports if you don't think they're ready yet. Even if they start later, they'll catch up soon.

NINE TO TEN

All sports can be introduced at these ages. Enthusiasm, desire for physical contact, and development of natural skills are characteristics of most kids during these years. Be prepared for intense interest in a role-model athlete: an older sibling, a nationally renowned sports star, a neighborhood athlete. Kids are also influenced by their young peers who are getting involved in baseball, soccer, karate, tennis, swimming, or whatever.

But they've also reached the ages when parents often begin urging and even pushing them to get into sports. If you find yourselves doing that, perhaps it's time to reread the recommendations on pages 31–34. Guide your youngsters to the sport or activity that fits them best. If they'd rather paint or play the violin, be willing to let go of any sports dreams you might have for them.

ELEVEN TO TWELVE

This is when sports may enter your child's life in a big way. At these ages, youngsters get started in real athletic competition. In almost every instance, those who eventually become outstanding competitors have started this early. Love of the game and hunger to play become ingrained, and the real skills begin to show. At this point in your child's sports development, it's a good idea to ask yourself about your own attitude: Are you focusing on your youngster's best interests or on your own sports fantasies for him/her?

THE TEENS

These are the years in which youngsters will become committed to a particular sport, because their advanced skills begin to pay off and their self-confidence grows. Your support for them is vital. You are off to many happy days of parenting—and don't forget to fill that scrapbook.

Of course, some teenage youngsters may decide they want to change to another sport or drop sports entirely. Make sure to let them know it's okay for them to make their own choices.

◆ Summing Up

There is no fixed age or magic formula for starting your youngsters off in sports. At the same time, there is no evidence that sports at an early age do any physical harm *if the activities are carefully supervised*. Emotional damage is harder to judge. You may think it's perfectly all right to direct your child into a sport at an early age, but listen to those about you who may see trouble: teachers, friends, and neighbors. Above all, don't close your mind with the statement, "I know what I'm doing."

◆ THE PARENT'S ROLE: WHAT SHOULD IT BE?

Hundreds of parents of young athletes have passed through my office. With the risk of oversimplification, I place them into three basic attitudinal groups, one that is constructive and two that can be troublesome:

1. Supportive Parents
2. Aggressive Parents
3. Reluctant Parents

◆ Supportive Parents

Supportive parents have a healthy attitude toward sports, and they try to instill that attitude in their kids. Their philosophy: you do your best, but learning is more important than winning, and the biggest benefit of sports is to enjoy them.

Although they may never have competed themselves, supportive parents are proud of their children's achievements in competition, and they offer encouragement freely and enthusiastically. They also understand the nature of injuries and their consequences, and have accepted the fact that to gain the values inherent in a sport, one must risk possible injury.

Supportive parents attend their children's games and practices when they can, and they listen receptively when their youngster replays the excitement of the day. They learn the sport and the rules of the sport. In short, they participate in every way.

But they don't get *over*involved. They don't push their kids and they don't interfere with the coaches who supervise their kids—unless they are concerned over lack of proper safety or injury-care procedures.

◆ Aggressive Parents

Aggressive parents push their kids. They may want their youngsters to fulfill their own youthful fantasies of being great athletes. They may envision being the parents of a young Olympian or a full-scholarship athlete. Or they may see future financial wealth as they read about the huge amounts of money made by professional athletes today, whether in football, baseball, basketball, tennis, golf, or other highly-paid spectator sports.

Parents who project their own fantasies and frustrations onto their children tend to berate them for making mistakes when they come home from a game—and sometimes right on the field in front of their teammates. Children in individual sports are put down when they lose, rather than being supported and comforted.

Aggressive parents are particularly poor in dealing with injuries. They cannot cope with the realities of a serious injury when it occurs. Their fanatical desire for a great athlete at all costs often blinds them to the damage caused by their attitude. How often have I had such a parent say to me: "I'm not pushing him, Doc, it's what he wants!" or "She can't be hurting *that* much!"

The case of one of my young patients illustrates the delusions that aggressive parents can have about their own children. Let's call her *Karen*. At the age of five, Karen was heavily involved in gymnastics, soccer, ballet, and swimming. I suggested to her parents that pushing her into all these activities was excessive and dangerous. They responded that they were not pressing her and she loved every minute of it. In reality, however, Karen was showing obvious signs of emotional distress. She was not participating in kindergarten group activities, was generally sulky, and kept hitting her younger brother. Eventually, I persuaded her parents to reconsider her rigorous sports schedule and their plans for her future.

Children like Karen may survive being pushed by their parents. But many never reach their peak. They burn out early and may develop strong resentments against their parents. The message here is that sports must be kept in proper perspective. They are but one aspect of life and should be balanced with the other important aspects, such as studies and family activities.

This doesn't mean you should not encourage discipline, consistent practice habits, and the best sports performance your children are capable of. That's being supportive. You want your kids to try their hardest. Just don't forget that they *are* kids.

◆   **Reluctant Parents**

These parents generally have no interest in competitive sports and they don't understand their children's interest in them. They may even have a negative attitude toward sports, possibly based on their own insecurities, which they transfer to their child. As a result, these parents have a high anxiety level about sports injuries. They are constantly telling their children, "You're going to get hurt, you're going to get hurt," and then when an injury occurs, "I told you you'd get hurt!" This, of course, is a good way to make the child feel guilty and increase the difficulty of medical care and recovery. There is nothing more trying for a competitive youngster in a contact/collision sport than to have to deal with this excessive parental anxiety.

Such parents need not have gotten themselves into this situation in the first place. If parents truly feel their child should not play high-risk sports, then guidance and direction should start long before the youngster picks up the ball or the hockey stick. Make these decisions about your children's sports activities well before things get to the point where the activities cannot be reversed without an emotional battle. Early on, the youngster should be directed towards noncontact sports: tennis, swimming, figure skating, running, golf, and the like.

If you tend to be a reluctant parent, you might also try to look at the situation from your youngster's point of view. Can you truly change the direction of a competitive youngster who is absolutely determined to play football or perform gymnastics? It's not likely without serious emotional damage. With some kids, it's just in their blood.

Another suggestion for reluctant parents (and *all* parents): *Learn as much as you can about the sport in which your child is participating.* You may find values in the sport you didn't know existed. Find out about the purpose of the sport, its rules and regulations, and its hazards. This knowledge can help you understand the sport and provide a perspective that will make you more supportive of your young athlete. For example, in my own family, my wife Estamarie was very fearful of our son Mark being involved in wrestling until she learned more about the sport and its character-building values.

◆   When There's a Conflict

In some families, of course, there will be a problem: The father may fall into one attitude category, while the mother falls into another. If you differ in the direction you feel your child should go and are openly divided on a specific sport, *don't allow the dissension to continue.* Work out a united family decision *before* your youngster begins participating in a sport. Both of you should be willing to consider compromises.

Single Parents

If you're a single parent in conflict over whether your child should enter a particular sport, don't try to go it alone. Talk to other single parents who have faced your situation and to people you trust for sound advice. You may need an objective "referee" to assist in resolving the problem: a sports physician, a coach, or a school counselor. Such experts can help you consider all the pros and cons and make a decision that both you and your child can live with comfortably. (Of course, two-parent families can profit from this counsel as well.)

3

A Parents' Guide to Sports Competition

◆

Thirteen-year-old *Tony* plays baseball in his neighborhood park. He's an outfielder on one of his community's eight Little League teams that play each other for the League championship.

Star quarterback *Jeff* has led his high-school football team to two straight state championships. He hopes to get an athletic scholarship to a major university and dreams of playing professional football.

At only fourteen, *Beth* is already a nationally ranked swimmer. She travels all over the country to perform in major competitive events and is aiming to break the national free-style record.

Tony, Jeff, and Beth represent just three of the many different levels of youth sports competition in the United States. If you have a child just starting out in sports, it's a good idea for you to familiarize yourself with the wide range of organized sports and what they require from both your children and you. Here's a rundown of the many varieties of sport and competition you may encounter.

◆   YOUTH-LEAGUE SPORTS

Youth-league sports consist of organized sports *outside* of school that sponsor local, regional, and often national competition. Millions of youngsters participate in these leagues, such as the Pop Warner Football League, the baseball Little League, and the Amateur Hockey Association. In the United States almost every sport—including soccer, basketball, wrestling, lacrosse, and martial arts—has a program for young athletes sponsored by a national organization. (You'll find a list of these organizations in the Appendix on page 347.) Many communities also sponsor organized youth sports teams—consult local officials for information.

Most youth-league sports programs are well organized and administered, with rules and regulations, safety standards, age standards, and formal playoff systems. However, in the name of winning there are sometimes violations— such as falsifying ages and weights of players—so parents of youngsters in these leagues should be vigilant in making sure that all regulations are being followed.

◆   Your Role As a Parent

If your child is going to be active in youth-league sports, your role should be to get involved and support your youngster. More specifically:

- Find out who runs the program and how it is organized.
- Learn what the sport is all about.
- Make sure your youngster is really interested.
- Know what the cost is in time and money.
- Show your support—for example, attend games as much as possible and keep your child's game schedule prominently displayed on the refrigerator door.
- Make sure that whenever possible the whole family attends important games.
- Set consistent rules for your youngster—before the season begins—on the performance of studies and household duties as required conditions for playing.

- Make sure your youngster is wearing good safety equipment (gloves, face mask, helmet, etc.).
- Monitor the safety of the playing facilities used by your youngster's team.
- Keep a scrapbook—it will be a source of smiles and chuckles years later (even when the score was horrendous!).

◆ Parents as Coaches—Good or Bad?

Many youth-league coaches are parents of participating youngsters. Is this a good idea? The answer depends on how the parent approaches coaching. There are good parent-coaches and then there are those who do a lot more harm than good.

The involvement of parents as coaches on youth teams *can* be invaluable. Kids are eager for adults to guide them; and if you have a good relationship with your own youngster, he or she will usually welcome you as a coach.

One reward of parent-coaching is the memories it builds up. The youngsters you've coached will enjoy recalling the funny things that happened when you came to practice, the big wins, and even the big losses. There's often in these memories a good deal of affection, which should give you much satisfaction.

So if you are a patient, supportive parent with insight into kids and a balanced perspective on youth sports, put on your glove or your soccer cleats, get down to the field, and sign up as a head coach or assistant coach. When you do get involved, be sure to follow the recommendations of the organization for that particular sport (see page 353 for a list of such organizations). Many of these organizations have helpful information for parent-coaches on such subjects as day-to-day organization, playing rules, safety procedures, and protective equipment.

◆ When Broader Competition Is Involved

Although many youth-league teams play only in their own local areas, some progress to regional competition—

and if they do well they may go on to sectional competition and even the national championships. There will be travel and expense, along with increased training, discipline, and pressure. The chances of being injured increase as well, because of fatigue, unfamiliar playing sites, and the tension of championship play.

What can you do to ease these problems if your youngster is involved in this expanded competition? Here are some guidelines:

- Keep a close eye on your youngster's well-being.
- Allow sufficient time for traveling.
- Try to maintain a positive, relaxed atmosphere.

Your youngster may have a chance to be in expanded competition, but you may not be able to afford the expense. If so, let your youngster know early on, before hopes are built up too high. On the other hand, be understanding if your youngster does *not* want to participate in regional or broader competition.

Some psychologists question the value of championship competition at these levels. But in my experience, the elite young athletes who participate in such competition are generally stable, self-confident youngsters who mature successfully.

◆   **INDIVIDUAL SPORTS**

In individual sports, solo performance is what counts rather than team play, although individual performers may be part of a team. Examples are gymnastics, swimming, tennis, and figure skating.

Qualitatively, individual sports are very different from team sports in several important ways. For one thing, children usually begin individual sports at very early ages—as young as three. For another, the training for an individual sport is far more rigorous and time-consuming than for a team sport. It is not unusual for this training to take up twenty or more hours a week. As a result, these children may become socially isolated from others in their age group. Training for the sport may be the dominant element in their lives.

Development in individual sports is a never-ending progression from one level of skill to the next, with increasing pressure at each level. The children who fail to progress drop out of the training system. On the other hand, if they continue to improve, their self-confidence builds. Eventually, these children will reach the elite category and require a full-time coach. Some may actually leave home to continue their training, living with the coach, a relative, or another family.

What gets youngsters hooked on individual sports? There's no clear-cut answer, but many youngsters have said that excelling in an individual sport gives them a "high" that nothing else does. What keeps them going is the feeling they get from doing a perfect arabesque in ballet or a triple jump in figure skating.

But to achieve this, they must be mature enough to accept the required discipline and sacrifice. They face constant pressure, severe limitations on social activity, and the possibility of serious injury. Small wonder that many drop out, especially during the early teens when the social sacrifices begin to be felt most keenly.

If you have a youngster in individual sports, be supportive rather than pressuring. Teach your youngster to take responsibility for his or her own body, to know its limitations, and to understand that serious overuse injuries can interrupt their training, sometimes for long periods.

◆ Parents Vs. Coaches

Although parents should get involved when their kids are active in individual sports, there's such a thing as getting *too* involved. You may think your *Betsy* is a potential Olympics champion in gymnastics, so you complain to her coach that she isn't getting enough instruction. Or you may want the coach to spend more time on certain aspects of the program.

My best advice is not to let your child become a pawn in a parent-coach conflict. A good coach usually knows how much potential a child may have in a particular sport. Your own opinion is understandably colored by parental pride, but it's wise to try for more objectivity. Very few children have the potential or drive to become tops in their sport. So unless your youngsters are among these few, don't insist that your coach push them. Their experience should be enjoyable, not painful.

◆ **When Your Child Wants Out**

Sometimes I get signals from the injured youngsters coming into my clinic that there's something wrong beyond their physical hurts. They may have a backache from gymnastics, a sore shoulder from swimming, or an aching knee from dancing. But their demeanor sends me a more serious message: *they want out.* They simply do not want to endure the rigorous disciplines required by their individual sport but are afraid to say so openly for fear of displeasing their parents.

If your child is involved in an individual sport, be alert for signs of a desire to quit. Reassure your child that it's okay to talk openly about this, and that there will be no punishment for dropping out. A child's emotional well-being is more important than sports glory.

◆ **National Ranking**

If your child achieves national ranking in an individual sport, your family will have to make some major adjustments. There's no way your young athlete can achieve success at this level without a total commitment, and that's going to mean sacrifice for the whole family.

Financial Pressure. Nationally ranked youngsters can put a big financial burden on their families. We've all heard of families that have mortgaged themselves into financial disaster for youngsters aspiring to Olympic positions, only to have it all fall apart in the end.

Sibling Sacrifice. The star athlete's brothers and sisters may be forced to give up some of their own educational opportunities or sports goals to further the star athlete's career. Needless to say, this can create some severe family problems.

Education. A nationally ranked athlete may not have time for a normal education. Where will that leave your youngster when the high-level sports competition is finished and it's time to go on to other pursuits? On the other hand, attempts to balance education and commitment to the sport may not work out.

What to Do?

Parents of nationally ranked athletes must be ready to deal with these difficulties. Fortunately, good counseling is available today in most sports centers. When you foresee your young athlete achieving this position, seek advice from professional experts. Then sit down with the whole family to discuss the options and the changes the future may bring.

◆ HIGH-SCHOOL SPORTS

The second major thrust of youth sports begins in high school. There's a big difference between high-school sports and the sports activities of younger years.

More Variety. Chances are your youngsters will already be active in some sports by the time they reach high school. But now they might want to explore new, unfamilar sports, and high schools offer a wide variety from which to choose. For the first time, your youngster may be able to try such sports as tennis, wrestling, gymnastics, track, and volleyball. Some schools may have more unusual sports like fencing.

More Sports Fever. In high-school sports, the drive for superiority and excellence grows more intense. Student athletes begin thinking seriously about championships and possible college athletic scholarships. In many high schools, sports dominate the school scene, sometimes at the expense of the academic side.

More Rules and Regulations. The school itself takes over many of the responsibilities you handled when your child was in youth-league sports. Rules and regulations imposed by the school and the state will deal with organization and discipline. The school coach assumes major responsibility for setting team standards.

◆ Your Role as a Parent

You may be saying to yourself, "Now that my youngster is in high school, I can relax and leave everything to the directors of the school sports program." Forget that thought. Particularly when it comes to the prevention and treatment of injuries, parents should take an active role. We'll deal with that role in detail in upcoming chapters. Remember, it's safety first.

◆ The State High School Athletic Association

Interscholastic competition between high schools is governed by a state athletic association, which establishes rules, regulations, and game schedules. Its goal is to maintain a competitive program that is coordinated, safe, and fair to all students.

Rules are usually developed by coaches, athletic directors, and principals, in line with national rules for each sport and recommendations by the sports medical committee and legal counsel.

◆ Important Rules You Should Know

To interact intelligently with your high-school sports program, you should familiarize yourself with the state association rules and regulations that govern it. Here are some typical rules, many of them related to injury prevention.

Transfer Rules

These rules govern the sports eligibility of students who transfer from one school district to another. Generally, the rules specify that the student is not eligible to play interscholastically at the new school until the beginning of the following school year.

Although transfer rules are sometimes challenged in court by parents of a young athlete, there are sound reasons for them. Parents of outstanding athletes have been known to move to a new town only because their youngster's athletic prowess will get more exposure in that town's high school. If this practice were to be allowed, high-school coaches might well start recruiting young athletes from neighboring or even distant cities, thus contributing to an overemphasis on high-school sports.

If your family is planning to move, learn about the transfer rules that apply to your new school. Then prepare your young athlete for any adjustment that will have to be made, so your child will understand why he or she must wait before playing. Also keep in mind that ignorance of the rule will not justify a waiver for your youngster.

Age Rules

Most sports medicine specialists, authorities on adolescence, and educators agree that no youngsters should be allowed to compete in high-school sports after the age of nineteen. Most rules specify that any student who turns nineteen on or before September 1 is ineligible to play that year. The reason: By that age, the athlete is far more physically developed than most of the other competitors, creating an imbalance that can lead to serious injuries.

Male-Female Rules

Most states have rules against coeducational teams in interscholastic high-school sports, although courts have overturned these rules in some states. From a sports medicine standpoint, there are very few high-school sports in which coed programs are desirable. They are definitely unacceptable in such sports as football, soccer, basketball, and baseball. With the male-female differences in body weight and muscular development, coed collision sports can result in serious injuries. And in limited-contact sports—such as volleyball, softball, and field hockey—the problem is that the boys almost totally dominate the teams. This robs the girls of their opportunity to excel in interscholastic high-school competition, and it also limits the number of girls who can participate.

Out-of-Season Practice Rules

These rules are designed to prevent some high schools from gaining unfair advantages over others by going in for intensive off-season practicing, training, and conditioning. All schools are required to pursue these activities under the same guidelines.

This doesn't mean that high-school athletes can't work out on their own during the summer. But if their coach is orchestrating these sessions, it's an infraction of the rules in many states.

Rules on School and Nonschool Competition

These rules regulate competition by high-school athletes outside of school. Some states forbid such activity totally—others may limit outside competition to one game and practice session during the season. Behind the rules are several objectives:

- To protect school athletes from overexertion that can damage their health
- To provide athletic participation for more students who do not play on school teams
- To promote the student-athlete's academic pursuits
- To prevent scheduling conflicts and problems arising from

involvement with different coaching and athletic philosophies

Make sure your own young athletes abide by the out-of-school rules in your locality. Be alert for signs of the "teenage overuse syndrome": irritability, poor eating, door slamming around the house. These are indications that your youngsters may be tiring themselves out by engaging in nonschool athletic activities on top of a demanding school athletic schedule. Not only is this detrimental to their health, it will leave them unable to perform at their best for their school team.

◆ The State System and You

These rules and others have been developed by state athletic associations to ensure the fairness and equity of high-school sports competition—and to keep an educationally sound balance between athletic and academic activities. To help further these objectives, it's wise for you as a parent to think twice before requesting a waiver to any of these rules on behalf of your own young high-school athlete. If you feel that a waiver is justified, present your request—but abide by the decision of the association, which will review it thoroughly. Unless the rules are strictly enforced and applied to all, the system will break down. Professionalism has already invaded college campuses; it should not be allowed in high-school sports.

4

The Young Athlete with Disability

◆

Participation by disabled youngsters is one of the fastest growing segments of youth sports. It was once taken for granted that physical disability or mental retardation ruled out sports activity. Now, however, it is widely accepted that disabled youngsters can not only participate in sports but can gain greatly in increased confidence and self-esteem. As a result of this change in attitude, sports programs for disabled youngsters are growing at a fast pace. As of 1991, there were about twenty-five national organizations throughout the United States developing community programs and sponsoring competition for disabled athletes of all ages. Probably the best known organization is the National Wheelchair Athletic Association, founded in 1956, which pioneered in establishing recreational and competitive sports for disabled people.

These organizations help to integrate disabled youngsters into the mainstream, regardless of their physical or mental limitations. Their participation in sports serves to reduce public prejudice and expand their freedom to join in normal activities. Sports are the great equalizer.

As an athletic surgeon, I have cared for a number of outstanding disabled athletes. One had cerebral palsy, yet played high-school football and now coaches. Others were a blind fencer, several paraplegics, and a young nationally-ranked skier with one leg. They are living proof that disabled youngsters can actively participate in sports.

Disabled youngsters are not necessarily interested in sports participation. But if your child does show enthusiasm for sports, your first step should be to identify the sports and then determine the feasibility of participation. The following pages briefly discuss various disabilities in terms of sports participation. For a comprehensive resource book, I recommend *Sports and Recreation for the Disabled: A Resource Manual*, by Michael J. Paciorek and Jeffery A. Jones (Indianapolis: Benchmark Press, 1989).

◆ PHYSICAL DISABILITIES

Six general types of physical disability are related to sports participation.

Loss of Limbs

Youngsters who are missing one or more limbs (either from amputation or a birth defect) can still participate in many sports. Today's sophisticated artificial legs make it possible to compete at a high level. Even youngsters who have lost both legs can participate in one of the many wheelchair competition programs.

Some of the most popular sports for youngsters missing limbs are skiing, basketball, track and field, soccer, tennis, and running.

Blindness

Partial or total blindness by no means rules out sports activity. Obviously, there is a wider selection for those youngsters who have some eyesight. But totally blind youngsters are active in many sports, including swimming and track and field.

Deafness

Partially or totally deaf youngsters can participate in all sports, although in certain sports special visual signals will have to be arranged. This is relatively simple and will enable your youngster to perform as well as any other. Consult the youth sports organization or the school coach for the sport in which your youngster is interested.

Cerebral Palsy

Cerebral palsy, usually related to brain damage in infancy, can result in muscles that are too tight or rigid, poor coordination of the arms and legs, and speech disturbances. However, many youngsters with cerebral palsy can participate in a variety of sports. In my own practice, I have cared for cerebral palsy youngsters playing football, tennis, soccer, and other school sports.

If you have a youngster with cerebral palsy who is interested in sports, discuss it with your physician.

Paraplegia

Paraplegia is paralysis from the waist down, either from a birth defect or an injury to the back or neck. Despite their disability, many paraplegics are intense competitors in sports ranging from ping pong to marathons. Basketball and track and field are other sports popular with paraplegics. International wheelchair games are held in these sports every year.

Injuries are frequent in some of the sports undertaken by these athletes, but are seldom serious. Most common are contusions, tendinitis, and blisters.

To get information about sports activity for your paraplegic youngster, call your state disability office and get in touch with the National Wheelchair Athletic Association and the National Handicapped Sports Association.

Other Disabling Conditions

Birth defects can include bone defects, weak or stiff joints, and inability to use certain muscles. Illnesses such as muscular dystrophy, *osteogensis imperfecta*, and Ehlers-Danlos Syndrome can cause disabling physical abnormalities. Any participation in sports activity depends on the severity of the problem, which should be determined by a physician.

◆ **MENTAL RETARDATION**

Mentally retarded youngsters (also known as "special needs" children) can participate in a wide variety of sports, depending on the severity of their disability.

Sports activities can be very important in helping a retarded youngster to feel accepted in his or her environment. The social interplay of these activities can reduce a feeling of isolation and bring about a healthy adjustment that will last into later years.

Ideally, kindergarten or even prekindergarten years are the best time to get a retarded youngster involved in group physical activity. The level of activity would depend on the potential of the child. Get as much guidance as possible from sources such as your physician, the child's therapist, and local agencies that assist special needs children.

Sports may not be recommended or may not be available for your youngster at an early age, but continue to pursue the possibility. As soon as sports become part of retarded youngsters' lives, their sense of belonging and self-esteem is enhanced. As they go on, their commitment to sports will become even stronger and their social adjustment easier.

Naturally, some retarded youngsters may not respond as positively to sports as others. They should not be forced into sports if it appears that they are not enthusiastic or will fail to benefit.

Many organizations sponsor programs for special needs children. One of the finest of these programs is the annual international Special Olympics. The number of volunteers who contribute their time and efforts to this and other programs for young disabled athletes is truly remarkable.

PART II

Reducing the Risks of
Sports Injuries

◆

5

Making Sure Your Child is Healthy

◆

Your eleven-year-old *Dave* wants to play Little League baseball. That's fine with you—baseball is a great game and Dave will surely enjoy Little League competition. You're ready to give him your blessings right now.

Not so fast. There's an important qualification that Dave must meet before you give your permission. *Dave must be healthy enough to play baseball.* That means he should undergo a pre-sport exam by a physician to make sure he has no physical or medical problems that would make it hazardous for him to play.

This is an essential first step in your *family sports safety program.* And it's smart to schedule a preseason physical every other year. Even if your youngster has already been active in sports, injuries or illness suffered after the initial preseason physical can be disqualifiers. Injury risks in sports are high enough; failing to take these precautions will make them even higher.

Why are pre-sport physicals so important? Consider the case of Gerald B., a fourteen-year-old high-school freshman who wanted to try out for the track team. During his pre-sport examination, the school physician took a thorough medical history that revealed that several members of Gerald's family had died prematurely of heart problems.

Based on this history, the doctor ordered tests of Gerald's heart. The results showed that Gerald had hypertrophic cardiomyopathy, a genetically transmitted enlargement of the heart. Because this condition is the leading cause of sudden death in young athletes, Gerald was disqualified for track and told he should not participate in any strenuous sports.

An extreme case perhaps, but it carries an important message for all parents: *Every child should have a complete medical evaluation before competing in a sport.*

◆   YOUR ROLE IN PRE-SPORT EXAMS

If your child is in school, the school physician or sports medical team will usually give the pre-sport physical. In individual sports, it's your responsibility to choose a physician to do the evaluation. All youth-league sports require a physical exam before a youngster may join the team, but again you have the responsibility for obtaining it.

When you are responsible for the exam, your first choice to do it should be a doctor who has your child's complete medical record, such as a pediatrician, a family physician, or a primary-care physician in an HMO.

If you don't have a regular doctor or medical insurance, you can take your child to a hospital clinic or local health center to obtain a pre-sport examination. If you need help in getting a pre-sport physical, call your state medical society or local hospital for assistance.

In addition to these sources for obtaining a pre-sport medical evaluation, many communities now have sports medical clinics that can provide such an exam. To locate the nearest sports medical clinic, call your state or county medical society.

There are some important things you can do to make sure that your youngster's pre-sport physical is as effective as possible.

◆ **Get a Complete Report**

Pre-sport medical exams should be as complete as possible. Otherwise, some conditions that can affect fitness for a sport—such as diabetes, ulcers, loose ligaments, and high blood pressure—will go undiscovered. The trouble is, when a doctor simply hands you a piece of stationery with the word "Normal" scribbled on it, you have no way of knowing whether or not the examination was thorough. To make sure the examination touches all the bases, ask your doctor to use one of the standard forms available for recording and reporting the results of pre-sport physical evaluations. You'll find recommended forms at the end of this chapter.

◆ **Give a Complete History**

Fourteen-year-old *Philip* reported to the sports clinic for a pre-season basketball physical. Fearing that he wouldn't be allowed to play, he didn't tell the doctor that he had epilepsy. He passed his physical. But even though he was taking medication, he had a violent, frightening seizure during a strenuous game. Fortunately, he recovered, but if he had revealed his epilepsy during the physical, the coach and trainer could have taken precautions to avoid any seizure.

When the doctor asks for a medical history, *nothing should be omitted*, including significant family medical history. It's better to provide too much information than too little.

In some situations, you may not be present during your youngster's exam. If you think that there are any conditions your youngster may fail to report for fear of being barred from play, inform the doctor about them in writing.

◆ **Monitor School Physicals**

For some school sports, you may be responsible for pre-sport exams, but most major team sports have annual "team

physicals" conducted by school personnel. Special exams are
required if the student has been injured or ill.

Don't relax simply because the school is conducting
your youngster's pre-sport physical. The quality of high-
school physicals can vary widely from thorough and comprehensive to hasty and superficial. In some cases, one team
doctor may spend an hour briefly examining fifty or sixty
students in the gym—not an ideal way to ensure that the
youngsters can perform safely in high-pressure sports.

So for your own peace of mind and the well-being of
your children, keep a close watch on how physicals are conducted in your school. Here's what you should look for:

The Ideal School Team Physical

A first-rate school physical should include four parts.
Privacy should be provided, since students will hesitate
to answer personal health questions frankly with other
teammates listening.

Coach's Exam: Here the student presents the coach with
the proper forms, completed and signed by the parent
or guardian. The coach then measures height and
weight and instructs the student on the procedures for
the rest of the exam.

Nurse's Exam: This station includes blood pressure,
medical history, eye exam, urine analysis, and blood
test. Because of the growing importance of nutrition in
sports health, the medical history should include a dietary record of the youngster's eating habits in and out
of the home.

Orthopedic Exam: The orthopedic exam should preferably be conducted by the certified trainer or orthopedic
physician who will be taking care of the team. However,
it may be done by the physical therapist or anyone
properly trained in joint examination who is familiar
with extremity and joint injuries and abnormalities.
This is a key exam and must be thorough. The examiner
should review any history of joint or extremity injuries
or surgery performed since the previous season, assess

the stability of all major joints, and record any laxity of these joints. Any youngsters with excess joint hypermobility or a history of serious joint injuries should be ruled ineligible to play.

Physician's Exam: In this final phase, the physician checks the student's medical history for completeness and accuracy, then performs a thorough medical examination that includes heart, lungs, lymph nodes, hernias, genitals, skin, and general well-being. The doctor indicates approval for competition on the student's record, for example with the phrase: "O.K. to go."

There is no national standard for physical examination forms used by high-school systems, although most state high-school organizations provide a recommended form. Find out what form your high school uses, and compare it for completeness with the recommended forms at the end of this chapter.

◆ A GUIDE TO MEDICAL CONDITIONS

What medical conditions should be considered when evaluating a youngster's fitness for sports? You should be familiar with these conditions in order to make sound decisions on whether your children should participate. The key question to ask yourself is: "What is best for my youngster?"

In the section that follows, we'll discuss the more common conditions to be considered, *some* of which can disqualify a youngster from sports competition. Keep in mind, however, that:

- Many of these conditions are not automatic disqualifications, but simply a reason for careful evaluation before making a decision.
- For the most part, these conditions permit *some* type of sports activity, depending on the severity of the condition.
- Medical reasons for disqualification differ in each major sports category—contact/collision, limited contact/impact,

and noncontact—and within the noncontact category there are differences among strenuous, moderately strenuous, and nonstrenuous sports.

- Our purpose here is to identify various conditions and comment on how they can affect sports activity. If your youngster has any of these conditions, you should get expert medical evaluation.

PHYSICAL IMMATURITY

Physical strength, size, and maturity are important factors in deciding whether a youngster is qualified to play in contact/collision sports such as football and lacrosse. A small, immature youngster playing football with much bigger, stronger youths is vulnerable to serious injury—and should be disqualified during the screening process. It's more important for players in contact/collision sports to be matched by developmental age than by chronological age. (For more guidance on this subject, see page 123.)

HEAD INJURIES

A history of severe head injury should eliminate your youngster from collision/contact sports. A good rule-of-thumb is that three or more concussions—even mild ones—should disqualify a player for at least the current season, and the youngster should be evaluated by a neurosurgeon before being permitted to play again.

Case in Point: A young football player in my care was addicted to the dangerous habit of spearing—that is, using his head as a battering ram against other players. In one season he suffered three concussions, one of which sent him to the hospital. On the very first play of the next year's opening football game he speared another player and went out like a light. I disqualified him for the season. This didn't sit well with his parents, who were hoping he'd win a football scholarship to college. But I believe that my decision saved him from a serious—possibly fatal—injury.

NECK INJURIES

Contact/collision and limited contact/impact sports are out for any youngster who has suffered previous neck (cervical spine) fractures, injuries to the spinal cord or major nerves to the arms and legs, or has certain congenital deformities. The final assessment should be made by a neurosurgeon or orthopedist.

Some youngsters have a *swan neck*, a long thin cervical spine that is vulnerable to injury. Other young people have structural abnormalities in their neck, which can be detected through X rays. The most common abnormality is two or three fused vertebrae, which could also cause neck instability and lead to injury. This might disqualify a youngster from contact/collision sports. Cine-radiographic X rays should be taken to look for neck instability.

EYES

Competition in contact/collision sports is not recommended for a youngster blind in one eye (that is, with less than 20/200 vision), and should be permitted only when special protective glasses are worn and parents have been warned about the risks of their youngster losing sight in the remaining eye through an injury. A player with only one good eye may be more vulnerable to injuries than one with normal vision. Most loss-of-eye injuries occur in ice hockey, and for a player already lacking vision in one eye this would mean total blindness. Poor two-eyed vision—20/40 or worse—can also disqualify youngsters from contact/collision sports unless they get special consent and wear corrective sport glasses.

HEARING LOSS

There is no reason to disqualify a youngster with hearing loss from any sport.

HEART DISORDERS

Every year sees sudden deaths among young players with heart conditions, so a decision on sports participation should be made only by a cardiologist. During a pre-sport physical exam, heart murmurs are the most common finding. The majority are functional murmurs—that is, sounds within a normal heart. But if there are *any* positive findings when the heart is checked during a pre-sport physical, a complete cardiac study should be carried out before a young person is allowed to participate in a strenuous sport.

ASTHMA

This is the most common condition related to breathing difficulty. Many asthmatics can participate in sports, but each asthmatic youngster's condition should be thoroughly evaluated by a specialist before permission is given to compete. A condition known as *exercise-induced asthma (EIA)* can often be controlled by medication so that the youngster can compete.

CYSTIC FIBROSIS

This is another breathing problem, caused by a congenital disorder. It does not necessarily limit sports activity—in fact, in 1991 a high-school basketball star with this condition played to the finals of his state championship. However, sports activity should be determined by the severity of the illness.

TUBERCULOSIS

This contagious disease is one pulmonary condition that will automatically disqualify a young athlete.

ALLERGIES

When the allergy is under control, either because of the season, the environment, or medication, a youngster can participate in sports. However, any required medication must always be on hand for emergency care during competition.

MONONUCLEOSIS

This is a viral infection characterized by fatigue, a sore throat, and general malaise. A youngster with these symptoms should be evaluated for this condition. One danger of participating in sports with mononucleosis is the possibility of an enlarged spleen which could be ruptured by a blow in a contact/collision sport. This injury can sometimes be fatal. When a pre-sports physical indicates the possibility of mononucleosis or an enlarged spleen, a blood test and a sonogram or spleen scan should be conducted. Permission to play should be granted only if these tests are normal.

HERNIAS

For the most part, hernias do not preclude participation in any sport. However, the severity of the hernia should be evaluated before permission to play is granted.

UNDESCENDED TESTICLE

No restrictions are needed for this condition.

KIDNEY

Any youngster with only one kidney should definitely be disqualified from collision sports.

SKIN CONDITIONS

These are usually treatable problems, such as boils, abscesses, and other contagious skin conditions. They may disqualify a youngster temporarily.

DIABETES

Although diabetes can be disqualifying, there are outstanding athletes with this condition. Each young diabetic must be evaluated individually to determine what sports may be permitted.

EPILEPSY

It is recognized today that an epileptic may participate in most sports. Generally, there is no restriction, but an epileptic subject to grand-mal seizures should probably not be active in contact/collision sports where head injuries can occur. Factors to be considered in permitting sports are the severity of the seizures, their frequency, and the amount of medication needed to control them. Coaches, trainers, and other responsible officials should be aware of the young athlete's condition and the medication required. Other athletes playing with the epileptic youngster should also be forewarned that a seizure is possible.

HYPERTENSION

Hypertension (abnormally high blood pressure) in youngsters is rarely severe enough to prohibit sports competition—in fact, exercise in proper amounts can actually help to lower blood pressure. However, the severity of the hypertension must be evaluated by a specialist, and any necessary treatment—such as dietary control or medication—must be instituted, with continuous monitoring.

CEREBRAL PALSY

Cerebral palsy and other neurological conditions must be judged on an individual basis. Ordinarily, these conditions will disqualify a youngster from contact/collision sports unless participation is approved by a neurologist. I know of at least one youngster with cerebral palsy who played high-school football successfully.

BACK PROBLEMS

If they are severe, several types of back problems can disqualify a youngster from sports competition:

Spondylolisthesis. A defect of the bones that support the frame of the vertebrae (see page 259 for more details).

Scoliosis. Curvature of the spine. All sports may be played with this condition unless the angle of deformity exceeds 30 degrees, in which case the decision should be based on the specific sport and the individual youngster. Severe scoliosis can be corrected by surgery, permitting most youngsters to play in less strenuous noncontact sports.

Scheuermann's Disease. An inflammatory condition affecting the growth centers of the spine. When this condition is found, it usually disqualifies a youngster for sports until the inflammation subsides and healing takes place. This can take from six months to three years.

Ruptured Discs. More common in young athletes than realized, and a condition frequently overlooked. Since ruptured discs heal, they are only a temporary disqualification. However, returning to a collision sport after rupturing a disc entails a high risk of continued back problems.

ORTHOPEDIC PROBLEMS

Orthopedic problems involve any parts of the body that move. Injuries to the arms and legs—the most frequent injuries in sports—can cause loss of stability or motion in the major joints severe enough to disqualify a young athlete from competition. Among the common orthopedic problems that can be disqualifying are:

Dislocating Shoulder. If the shoulder dislocates readily, the youngster should not be allowed to compete until the condition is corrected through surgery. (See page 213 for more on this condition.)

Unhealed Fracture. Any fracture that has not properly healed should disqualify a young athlete until the condition is corrected.

Knee Instability. Every knee injury must be judged individually. Serious knee injuries may eliminate a youngster from sports requiring high speed and agility. However, some athletes have been able to compete in spite of torn knee ligaments. *Best advice*: Follow your surgeon's recommendations.

HEMOPHILIA

Contact/collision sports are usually not recommended for youngsters with this hereditary condition. Permission to play in other sports should be based on a consultation with a pediatrician and a hematologist. It would depend on the type and severity of the bleeding tendency.

SICKLE CELL ANEMIA

Another hereditary blood disease, this one primarily afflicts blacks. Although it is no longer considered a disqualifier for contact/collision sports, the condition should be monitored carefully by a physician.

◆ HANDLING MEDICAL DISQUALIFICATION

Your fourteen-year-old *Bob* wants to try out for his high-school football team. During the team physical, the examining physican notes that last year Bob's knee ligaments were injured in an automobile accident. The physician wants Bob examined by an orthopedic specialist before giving him an okay to play football.

After examining Bob, the specialist explains that Bob should not play football because his knee ligaments have never healed properly. Although this condition does not affect his normal activities, playing football would make his leg vulnerable to more serious injury.

After receiving the orthopedist's report, the team physician disqualifies Bob from playing football. This is a tough blow for Bob, as it would be for any teenager. How you and the team physician deal with his rejection will be critical to his confidence and self-esteem.

Explain the Reasons Fully. The team physician should give Bob a complete explanation of why he cannot play football. This won't make him feel any better, but at least he'll know that the decision was in his best interests.

Give Support. Let Bob know you're proud of him and

that he has no reason to feel ashamed about his disqualification.

Find Alternatives. Don't let Bob sit around brooding over his rejection. Try to get him interested in another sport that would not be a risk to his knee. The coach can reassure the youngster that he's still needed by offering him a sideline position such as team manager or equipment manager.

◆ Seeking a Medical Waiver

The physician in your daughter *Sharon*'s high school has just barred her from playing field hockey because she has diabetes. You feel that since her condition is controlled through medication, she should be able to play without risk—and Sharon's physician agrees.

Your option is to request a medical waiver. How you do this depends on the procedures of your state's athletic association, which will decide if the waiver should be granted. The school principal or athletic director will advise you how to proceed. In most cases, you would submit a letter to the association from Sharon's doctor saying that she is qualified to participate and specifying any restrictions, dangers, or precautions. The association will review your request and make a decision.

◆ SAMPLE FORMS

The following two forms are recommended by the American Academy of Pediatrics for use in preparticipation physical exams.

SPORTS PARTICIPATION HEALTH RECORD

This evaluation is only to determine readiness for sports participation. It should not be used as a substitute for regular health maintenance examinations.

NAME _____ AGE _____ (YRS) GRADE _____ DATE _____

ADDRESS _____ PHONE _____

SPORTS _____

The Health History (Part A) and Physical Examination (Part C) sections must both be completed, at least every 24 months, before sports participation. The Interim Health History section (Part B) needs to be completed at least annually.

PART A — HEALTH HISTORY:
To be completed by athlete and parent

	YES	NO
1 Have you ever had an illness that:		
a. required you to stay in the hospital?		
b. lasted longer than a week?		
c. caused you to miss 3 days of practice or a competition?		
d. is related to allergies? (ie, hay fever, hives, asthma, insect stings)		
e. required an operation?		
f. is chronic? (ie, asthma, diabetes, etc)		
2 Have you ever had an injury that:		
a. required you to go to an emergency room or see a doctor?		
b. required you to stay in the hospital?		
c. required x-rays?		
d. caused you to miss 3 days of practice or a competition?		
e. required an operation?		
3 Do you take any medication or pills?		
4 Have any members of your family under age 50 had a heart attack, heart problem, or died unexpectedly?		
5 Have you ever:		
a. been dizzy or passed out during or after exercise?		
b. been unconscious or had a concussion?		
6 Are you unable to run 1/2 mile (2 times around the track) without stopping?		
7 Do you:		
a. wear glasses or contacts?		
b. wear dental bridges, plates, or braces?		
8 Have you ever had a heart murmur, high blood pressure, or a heart abnormality?		
9 Do you have any allergies to any medicine?		
10 Are you missing a kidney?		

11 When was your last tetanus booster? _____

12 For Women
a. At what age did you experience your first menstrual period? _____
b. In the last year, what is the longest time you have gone between periods? _____

EXPLAIN ANY "YES" ANSWERS _____
_____
_____

I hereby state that, to the best of my knowledge, my answers to the above questions are correct.

Date _____

Signature of athlete _____

Signature of parent _____

PART B — INTERIM HEALTH HISTORY:
This form should be used during the interval between preparticipation evaluations. Positive responses should prompt a medical evaluation.

1. Over the next 12 months, I wish to participate in the following sports:
a. _____
b. _____
c. _____
d. _____

2. Have you missed more than 3 consecutive days of participation in usual activities because of an injury this past year?
Yes _____ No _____
If yes, please indicate:
a. Site of injury _____
b. Type of injury _____

3. Have you missed more than 5 consecutive days of participation in usual activities because of an illness, or have you had a medical illness diagnosed that has not been resolved in this past year?
Yes _____ No _____
If yes, please indicate:
a. Type of illness _____

4. Have you had a seizure, concussion or been unconscious for any reason in the last year?
Yes _____ No _____

5. Have you had surgery or been hospitalized in this past year?
Yes _____ No _____
If yes, please indicate:
a. Reason for hospitalization _____
b. Type of surgery _____

6. List all medications you are presently taking and what condition the medication is for.
a. _____
b. _____
c. _____

7. Are you worried about any problem or condition at this time?
Yes _____ No _____
If yes, please explain: _____
_____
_____

I hereby state that, to the best of my knowledge, my answers to the above questions are correct.

Date _____

Signature of athlete _____

Signature of parent _____

Part C – PHYSICAL EXAMINATION RECORD

NAME _____ DATE _____ AGE _____ BIRTHDATE _____

Height _____   Vision: R _____/_____, corrected _____, uncorrected _____

Weight _____   L _____/_____, corrected _____, uncorrected _____

Pulse   _____   Blood Pressure _____ Percent Body Fat (optional) _____

	Normal	Abnormal Findings	Initials
1. Eyes			
2. Ears, Nose, Throat			
3. Mouth & Teeth			
4. Neck			
5. Cardiovascular			
6. Chest and Lungs			
7. Abdomen			
8. Skin			
9. Genitalia - Hernia (male)			
10. Musculoskeletal: ROM, strength, etc.			
a. neck			
b. spine			
c. shoulders			
d. arms/hands			
e. hips			
f. thighs			
g. knees			
h. ankles			
i. feet			
11. Neuromuscular			
12. Physical Maturity (Tanner Stage)	1. 2. 3. 4. 5.		

Comments re: Abnormal Findings: _____

_____

_____

_____

PARTICIPATION RECOMMENDATIONS:

1. No participation in: _____

_____

2. Limited participation in: _____

_____

3. Requires: _____

_____

4. Full participation in: _____

Physician Signature _____

Telephone Number _____ Address _____

American Academy of Pediatrics   ©Copyright 1990 HE0086

6

Five Special Medical
Considerations

◆

The healthier a young athlete the less risk of sports injuries. Guidelines in this chapter cover five important health areas that often generate controversy in the households of young athletes:

- Nutrition and diet
- Drugs and the young athlete
- The young female athlete
- Wrestling and weight control
- Weight lifting and the growing body

◆ **NUTRITION AND DIET:
EATING AND COMPETING**

You may not think of nutrition and diet as important factors in preventing sports injuries, but consider this: Good eating habits can improve your young athlete's fitness, strength, and performance—all of which contribute to avoiding injuries. Sports medical experts are putting more and more emphasis on nutrition as an important factor in keeping a young athlete in top condition.

But how do you control your young athlete's diet? With very young athletes it's not that much of a problem, because they're under constant supervision. But with teenage athletes it's a different story—their eating habits are not easily controlled. In many households both parents work or a single parent works, so mealtimes may be irregular and the youngsters left on their own in the kitchen. Although a good diet should be important to these young athletes, they'll usually ignore it unless they are extremely well motivated to keep themselves healthy for competition and development. Their diet will often consist of anything that tastes good and is convenient, regardless of its nutritional value.

So the task of instilling good eating habits in your teenage athlete can be formidable. One way to make it easier is to catch youngsters early—if you get them used to low-fat, low-cholesterol foods before they're ten, they will not be so likely to live on junk food when they reach their teens.

As much as possible, try to provide an organized pattern of meals at home. Find at least one meal during the day—whether breakfast or dinner—where everyone sits down and eats together. The benefits are abundant, both nutritionally and psychologically.

Although poor nutrition can exist in any family, it is most prevalent in low-income homes. Athletic coaches and trainers should be aware of this problem and try to provide families with information and sources of assistance. Every coach and trainer should be able to give parents an information sheet with basic guidelines for a balanced diet and recommended reading on nutrition.

◆ Guidelines for a Young Athlete's Diet

Most sports nutritionists recommend a high-carbohydrate (at least 60 percent), low-fat (15 percent), and moderate-protein (25 percent) diet for young athletes. Although there is no scientific proof that a high-carbohydrate diet improves performance, sports nutritionists recommend it because carbohydrates are the best and most efficient fuel for the young body. They are easily broken down in the body and utilized by the muscles.

Any diet that parents plan for their young athletes should include the four basic food groups:

Milk. Although not complete, this essential food, as well as milk products such as cheese and yogurt, adds much to the growing body: calcium, protein, vitamin D, and minerals. Three to four cups of skim milk a day are recommended.

Carbohydrates. Supplied by pasta, cereal, bread, crackers, corn, rice, flour, potatoes, peas, squash, and lima beans.

Fruits and Vegetables. Essential foods that supply minerals, vitamins, and fiber. Fruit and vegetable juices also supply these nutrients.

Meats and Fish. Both supply high amounts of protein, especially fish, which is high on the recommended list of daily foods.

Since teenagers tend to snack, it's a good idea to have a variety of snack foods on hand that are not just empty calories. Try fruit, popcorn, pizza, nonfat fruit yogurt, cut-up raw vegetables, low-fat puddings, bagels, ginger snaps, low-fat crackers, and fruit popsicles.

More Food Tips

Avoid excessive salt and saturated fats such as butter, beef, pork, and ice cream. One way to do this is to serve more ethnic foods, many of which provide more fiber, less salt and fat, and more fruits and vegetables than the typical U.S. diet. Examples are Chinese stir-fry dishes, Italian pasta dishes, and Mexican tortillas.

Although organic foods may not have added nutritional value, their advantage is freedom from preservatives.

For additional guidance on good nutrition for your young athletes, two reference books can be useful:

- *The Athlete's Kitchen* by Nancy Clark (New York: Bantam Books, 1986).
- *Eat to Compete* by Marilyn and Keith Peterson (Chicago: Yearbook Medical Publishers, 1988).

Checking Up

Using the preceding guidelines, it's a good idea to appraise the nutritional content of family meals periodically. Keep a detailed list of all foods eaten or purchased over the course of a week. Review it for quality and balance and make any changes needed to improve it. You might want to show it to the nutritionist in your local hospital.

◆ **The Pregame Meal**

Some sports nutritionists maintain that a high-carbohydrate diet for two or three days before a competitive event can "load" the body with extra energy. However, there is little evidence that this is true for adolescent athletes. The most important nutritional benefit comes from a steady, balanced diet week in and week out.

But the last meal before a game *can* significantly affect the young athlete's performance and vulnerability to injury. Both the timing of the meal and its ingredients are important.

Recommendations:

- Make sure the meal is eaten at least two-and-one-half hours before the competitive event. One's body cannot do two things well at once, and if it's busy digesting food it can't also be running a 100-yard dash or playing a strenuous soccer game.
- Don't let your youngster eat too much or too little. This amount will vary with individual teenage chemistry, and you will have to determine your youngster's response to eating and competing through experience. Anxieties, pressures, and pregame emotional outbursts can burn off calories and leave youngsters hungry during competition.
- Don't go for the outmoded high protein, "steak before the game" meal—it's not physiologically beneficial for either high performance or good health. Modest portions of carbohydrates such as pasta are best. Don't force your youngster to eat more than is wanted.

- Try to pick foods that your young athlete enjoys, not has to force down.
- There is no agreement by nutritionists on the value of eating candy shortly before competition. Although the sugar can provide a quick energy boost, some nutritionists believe this is followed by a steep drop in energy that can reduce performance.

◆   **Water, Water, Water**

Dehydration—that is, loss of body water—is probably the greatest health threat to young athletes during any sports competition. In fact, it can be life threatening (see section on heat stroke, page 135). Many young athletes don't realize that thirst can be a very late indicator of dehydration—by the time they are thirsty, they may already be in trouble.

Guidelines:

- Water must always be available during a competitive event or practice session—*without exception.*
- Water can be taken freely without worry.
- Cold water is more rapidly ingested than warm, and helps to control body temperature.
- Special electrolyte drinks are not necessary—water provides the same benefits for a lot less money.
- Water is more important during a game than salt replacement—in fact, sports medical experts no longer recommend salt tablets before and during a game, because they do not break up rapidly enough in the stomach to supply the necessary salt replacement.

◆   **DRUGS AND THE YOUNG ATHLETE**

The use of drugs to improve athletic performance is unhealthy and dangerous—and many are illegal or banned for sports use. They have no place in the world of the athlete, and cause serious side effects and poor judgment that can

---

Nutrition Checklist for Parents

1. *Make sure the family eats together at least once a day.*
2. *Always have nutritional foods available in the refrigerator and pantry.*
3. *List everything your young athlete eats during one week and review its nutritional value.*
4. *Have your athlete eat a good carbohydrate meal at least two-and-one-half hours before game time.*
5. *Tell your youngster to drink plenty of water during training and playing.*
6. *Bring brownies, cookies, or other "life-support" foods with you to the games—they make the best recovery medicine, win or lose.*

---

result in unnecesary injuries. As a parent, you can do much to steer your young athletes away from dependence on chemical support that could ruin their future.

There is no scientific proof that any drugs improve the level of athletic performance (the only exception being anabolic steroids). Unfortunately, however, a large number of athletes use drugs. As a parent, you should be aware of the problem and what steps you can take to deal with it.

Recommendations:

- Insist that the team coach make a positive statement—orally and in writing—about drug-free sports both to the young athletes and their parents.
- Make sure there are adequate rules on drug use. Any young athlete using drugs should be "benched" immediately until use is stopped and therapy instituted. However, with a first offense, it's preferable to keep the youngster on the team where the parents and coach can monitor the problem together. Kicking the athlete off the team can be a psychological blow that could lead to more drug abuse.

- If there's a second offense, the young athlete should immediately be dismised from the team.
- Make it clear to team officials that any coach who suggests that an athlete use drugs should be summarily dismissed.
- Make sure your young athlete knows both the school regulations and the state athletic association regulations concerning drugs.
- As a parent, learn all you can about drugs, responses to drugs, and how to recognize drug use (for warning signs, continue on in this section).
- Discourage excessive use of vitamins, amino acids, and protein compounds.

What about drug testing in high schools? It can be a deterrent to drug use by young athletes. However, mandatory testing is exorbitantly expensive and involves unsettled legal issues. Some schools are using a voluntary, random testing program. Such a program can exert social pressure on youngsters to be "clean."

◆   Parents' Guide to Drugs

When talking to parents and young athletes about drugs, I divide them into four categories: *uppers, downers, builders, and cures.* Some of these drugs are taken for recreational purposes, some to improve sports performance, and some to ease the pain of injuries.

Uppers

In sports, uppers are used to increase endurance and speed, although there is no solid evidence that they do so. Their primary effect is to stimulate a "high." Uppers are dangerous drugs that have caused deaths of several outstanding athletes and have been responsible for the loss of gold medals in Olympic competition. The most commonly used uppers are:

How to Recognize Drug Abuse

You may start with a gut feeling that something is not right with your youngster. If you suspect drugs, look for these specific signs:

1. *Glassy look, bloodshot eyes, dilated pupils.*
2. *Weight loss, paleness, sloppy appearance.*
3. *Change in appetite—sharp increase could mean marijuana use, while decrease is symptomatic of cocaine or crack use.*
4. *Slight slur in speech, word mix-up.*
5. *Runny, stuffy nose or regular nosebleeds (indicates possible cocaine use).*
6. *Poor gait, rapid breathing even at rest.*
7. *Chronic lack of sleep or abnormal sleep pattern.*
8. *Slow response, weak concentration.*
9. *Reduced motivation, poor school performance.*
10. *Personality change: aggressiveness, depression, nervousness, restlessness, agitation.*
11. *Tell-tale drug equipment in room or basement: cigarette rolling paper, spoons, deodorizers, glass vials, single-edge razor blades, small locked boxes, plastic baggies.*

COCAINE

A widely used drug, cocaine is a potent, toxic stimulant that produces euphoria followed by depression followed by a craving for more cocaine.

Cocaine overstimulates the nervous system, increases blood pressure, and forces a faster heartbeat. An overdose can cause convulsions within thirty to sixty seconds after use, and death can follow immediately. Crack is the freebase or raw form of cocaine. Cocaine is extremely addictive and it is dangerous to try it even once.

AMPHETAMINES

These are potent chemical stimulants marketed by prescription under such brand names as Benzedrine and Dexadrene. They give a false sense of security by masking fatigue—and contrary to the impressions of athletes who use them, they do not improve timing, endurance, performance, or speed. In their freebase form, amphetamines are extremely addicting and can cause hallucinations when toxic amounts accumulate in the body. Several international bicycle racers have died from using amphetamines.

MARIJUANA

Appears to be mild and relatively harmless, but it is actually harmful and deceitful. Despite giving a sense of well-being, it impairs short-term memory, sense of timing, concentration, and coordination. It also may lead to the use of heavy drugs. However, marijuana does not kill, and there is no evidence that it leaves permanent effects.

NICOTINE

Nicotine—the major drug in tobacco—is well known for its devastating long-term effects: cancer, heart disorders, and lung diseases. Less known are its serious short-term effects when used by athletes during competition: rapid pulse, increased blood pressure, shortness of breath, and excessive sweating—all of which erode performance.

Although smoking is now less socially acceptable than in the past, its dangers are still largely disregarded by school-age athletes. And many young athletes emulate their professional sports heroes by using chewing tobacco, which can cause cancer of the mouth. If your youngster must chew something during competition, let it be bubble gum.

CAFFEINE

Caffeine is acceptable in moderation. But caffeine in doses over fifteen milligrams (five to six cups of coffee) is prohibited by the International Olympic Committee (IOC). It can then have significant side effects, such as an increased heart rate, higher blood pressure, irregular heart rhythm, diuretic effects, insomnia, anxiety, and irritability. Caffeine should be taken in moderation whether in the form of coffee or cola drinks.

Downers

Downers—also called depressants—are used to quiet the nerves or induce sleep. They are all dangerous and do not benefit an athlete's performance—to the contrary, they can cause confusion and loss of concentration. Moreover, depressants are dependency drugs with serious withdrawal symptoms: anxiety, headaches, insomnia, and sometimes tremors.

Use of downers can be recognized by slurred speech, irrational thinking, poor judgment, and the appearance of drunkenness. The major downers are:

BARBITURATES

Prescription drugs with brand names such as Seconal, Nembutal, and Phenobarbital, they are used primarily to relax or induce sleep. Known on the street as "barbs" or "reds," these drugs are usually taken as pills or capsules. When present in the system during competition, they leave an athlete unable to respond with agility and speed. They cause depression and can be fatal when combined with alcohol.

TRANQUILIZERS

Although chemically different from barbiturates, these habit-forming prescription drugs are also used to reduce tension. Improperly used, they can be mentally and physically debilitating. A teenager should rarely require tranquilizers, and in those few cases should take them only when prescribed by a reputable doctor. Unfortunately, they are widely available on the street.

ALCOHOL

A habit-forming depressant, it slows down all physical functions and interferes with judgment and self-control. Although young athletes seldom drink during a game, they frequently abuse alcohol afterwards—as a post-game "thirst quencher." The earlier these kids start drinking, the greater the chances they'll become alcoholics. It cannot be emphasized too strongly that young athletes *should not drink.*

Builders

These drugs are used in sports to increase performance, strength, and muscle mass.

ANABOLIC STEROIDS

Known in athletics as "the sauce," steroids are widely used throughout the sports world despite being illegal. Although steroids definitely build strength and muscle mass, their effect on performance was not accepted until the Canadian runner Ben Johnson broke the 100-meter sprint world record in the 1988 Olympics after prolonged steroid use. He was later stripped of his gold medal by the IOC. Unfortunately, use of steroids by high-school athletes has increased in the years since.

If you think steroids are safe, consider these potential effects:

- In some cases, death
- Closing the growth centers early and stunting growth in the teenager
- Atrophy of testicles and possible sterility
- Liver damage and hepatitis
- Damage to heart muscles that can be fatal

Tip-Offs to Steroid Use

1. *Increased acne during lifting program.*
2. *Personality changes, particularly increased agitation or temper tantrums.*
3. *Rapid increase in size and shape of muscles, particularly arms and shoulders.*
4. *Your youngster is working out at a commercial gym that specializes in heavy lifting and massive body development.*

- Psychological effects (personality changes, aggressiveness, temper tantrums)
- Acne
- Irreversible baldness
- Specifically in females: mustache, beard, husky male voice, grossly large clitoris (irreversible)

This list should put you on guard against any use of steroids by your young athletes.

PROTEINS AND AMINO ACIDS

Like steroids, protein and amino acid compounds are used to build bigger, stronger bodies. They are perfectly legal and widely available in gyms, fitness centers, health stores, and sports equipment centers. The compounds are sold in all forms from powders to pills.

The advertising for these compounds is misleading. Although they won't do any harm, there is no evidence that they will make a growing body bigger and stronger, so it is totally unnecessary for any young athlete to spend money on them.

Cures

These therapeutic drugs are used to help heal injuries or improve the athlete's health. Some are available only by prescription, and some are banned in competition. To find out if any particular drug is banned for athletic competition, call the United States Olympic Committee hotline (1-800-233-0393).

DMSO

A popular name for *dimethyl sulfoxide*, the most controversial of all quick-cure liniments. Liniments in general have a beneficial effect on sore muscles, bruises, aches, and pains (as do massages and ice). But DMSO is different because it actually penetrates the body, even leaving a garlic-like taste on the tongue after being applied to the skin. Although DMSO is beneficial to the sore area, it may also be hazardous, since it is a petroleum chemical that circulates through the body. As yet, no conclusive studies are available on possible side effects, and I do not recommend its use until research is completed. Meanwhile, several other liniments work just as well, including wintergreen, Ben Gay, and Liquid Ice.

ANTI-INFLAMMATORY DRUGS

These drugs are used to reduce pain and swelling caused by injuries or overuse. Some are commonly used over-the-counter drugs such as aspirin and ibuprofen and prescription drugs such as phenylbutazone, indomethacin, and naprolene.

Anti-inflammatory drugs are not dangerous; they do not cause dependency and psychophysical damage as do cocaine and other heavy drugs. Nevertheless, over-the-counter anti-inflammatory drugs should be used in moderation—even aspirin. When taken in large amounts for long periods, these drugs can produce serious side effects. The strong prescription types should not be used by the teenage athlete except in unusual circumstances and with careful monitoring.

ANTIHISTAMINES-DECONGESTANTS-COUGH SYRUPS
These medications are used for allergies, colds, and pulmonary conditions such as asthma, hay fever, and bronchitis. Although they may be perfectly good medications, some are banned for athletic competition.

PAIN KILLERS
Over-the-counter pain killers such as aspirin are perfectly acceptable. But if young athletes require stronger prescription pain killers, I believe they should not be playing.

A note about birth control pills: There is no ban on the use of oral contraceptives during athletic competition, although one type of birth control pill was banned until 1988.

◆ What About Vitamins?

Though not truly drugs, vitamins are used so excessively in sports that they qualify for discussion under chemical abuse. Vitamins taken in doses larger than the U.S. Recommended Daily Allowance (RDA) have not demonstrated any increase in athletic strength, endurance, or performance. Moreover, overusing them can produce dangerous side effects, such as:

- *Vitamin A*: Vomiting, fatigue, lethargy, hair loss, and liver disease
- *Vitamin D*: Headaches, muscle stiffness, weakness, kidney stones, and excessive thirst
- *Vitamin E*: Nausea and fatigue
- *Vitamin C*: Diarrhea and kidney stones

Vitamins should be used only in cases of vitamin deficiency or special medical problems diagnosed by a physician. Current data suggest that vitamin supplements are unnecessary for the young athlete eating a balanced diet.

Unfortunately, heavy advertising of vitamins tends to promote their overuse.

Recommendation: If you think your young athlete is consuming overdoses of vitamins, get your doctor's advice and find out who, if anyone, recommended the vitamins to your youngster. If you think your athlete is undernourished or dehydrated, consult your physician, a nutritionist in your local hospital, or both to find out if there might be a vitamin deficiency.

◆ THE YOUNG FEMALE ATHLETE

Since the 1970s, females' participation in sports competition has increased dramatically. So has their athletic performance—compared with men in the same sports, their times and skills have improved at a 10 to 15 percent higher rate than those of their male counterparts. Women's ability to excel in athletics is now widely recognized. They are increasing their endurance (marathons), their strength (swimming, field events), and their skills (tennis, soccer, volleyball, skiing). The once unusual stories of such women as Babe Didrikson Zaharias (a phenomenal all-around female athlete who won two Olympic Gold Medals in track and field and was twice U.S. Women's Golf Champion) are now becoming commonplace.

Along with these accomplishments has come a corresponding increase in self-confidence. Female athletes have successfully destroyed the myths that they will become overdeveloped and muscle-bound and lose their femininity.

◆ Are There "Female" Sports Injuries?

The answer is no, with one exception: blows to the breast. And such blows are not a major concern—there is no evidence that they can cause cancer or other problems. However, female athletes should wear protective sports bras to give support and prevent severe contusions.

In two sports—field hockey and basketball—females

are incurring an increasing number of serious knee injuries. These are usually *anterior cruciate ligament* ruptures (see page 308 for more information) that occur in powerful, fast, field-hockey players and in tall, athletic, basketball players. In high-school competition, female basketball players suffer a higher percentage of all kinds of injuries than male players.

Shoulder injuries and cartilage tears of the knee are less frequent in young females than in young males, while kneecap dislocations and kneecap stress injuries are *more* frequent (because of a difference in pelvic structure). There is no difference in the frequency of shin splints, stress fractures, and ankle injuries.

◆ Iron-Deficiency Anemia

Female susceptibility to iron-deficiency anemia can be a problem in sports, because iron in the blood cells helps to carry oxygen, and this combination of iron and oxygen provides much of the energy needed to run and compete.

In girls, iron deficiency may be indicated by excessive menstrual flow, listlessness, and pallor. By all means, if this happens with your young athlete, have her iron level checked by a physician, who may prescribe iron supplements. Such foods as liver, prune juice, raisins, dried apricots, baked beans, and spinach provide iron.

◆ Menstruation

Having a period should not interfere with exercise or sports competition. Although excessive flow or cramps may trouble some young athletes, there's no reason why they shouldn't compete if they want to.

During prolonged strenuous training and competition, such as in distance running, irregular flow or absence of a period (amenorrhea) is not uncommon. This condition is neither serious nor abnormal. However, to reassure both you and your youngster, it's a good idea to consult a doctor when there's any menstrual irregularity.

◆   **Eating Disorders**

Two serious eating illnesses can stem from the psychological problems of adolescent girls: *anorexia nervosa* and *bulimia.*

Anorexia Nervosa

Anorexia nervosa is an emotional disorder characterized by abnormal loss of weight from excessive dieting and loss of appetite. This illness can be triggered by family conflicts, such as a girl's need to control her own life to thwart overbearing parents. Emotional insecurity and a reluctance to enter sexual maturity may also lead to anorexia nervosa. Whatever the cause, it is a serious, even dangerous illness that in extreme cases can be fatal. Obviously, it can weaken young female athletes to the point where they are very vulnerable to injuries.

Anorexia nervosa often goes unrecognized until serious damage is done. Be alert for lack of appetite, weight loss, lethargy, and withdrawal. If you see these signs, seek professional advice immediately—it is better to appear overcautious than to catch serious problems too late.

Bulimia

Bulimia is a similar disorder, characterized by loss of weight through deliberate vomiting after eating. Teenage youngsters with this problem may consume and vomit a whole meal several times a day. Though not as serious as anorexia nervosa, bulimia also requires medical attention.

◆   **WRESTLING AND WEIGHT CONTROL**

Wrestling is not only the oldest sport in the world, it is one of the fastest growing sports in the United States. As of 1991, there were half a million young wrestlers in competition. If you have a young wrestler in your family, you may not know as much as you should about "making weight." Most books on sports injuries have little practical advice for parents on dealing with weight loss when it becomes a problem.

Weight reduction can be a planned strategy for achieving competitive superiority in wrestling competition. The objective is to wrestle in the best possible weight class at which the wrestler still has his full strength. However, weight reduction can be carried too far, to the point when a young wrestler goes below his acceptable weight level and starts losing strength and endurance.

Members of the sports medical community are deeply concerned about unhealthy weight loss in young wrestlers, not only because of the loss of strength and endurance, but also because the young athlete becomes depressed and loses the ability to concentrate, thus affecting classroom performance.

◆ What's Behind the Problem?

Basically, that excessive weight loss is not treated as a sports injury, as it should be. Many coaches continue to use improper methods for weight control, even though they have safe, medically recommended formulas available to them. Parents are usually unaware of the weight-loss program a coach is using.

There's nothing wrong with weight loss within an acceptable limit: around 7 percent of body weight. In fact, controlled weight loss can significantly improve wrestling performance.

Excessive weight loss is a different matter. Although no medical evidence shows that it does permanent damage, it can produce serious short-term effects. Academic studies may suffer through inability to concentrate because of hunger, thirst, and restlessness. In competition, the young wrestler may be handicapped by slow body responses and general weakness.

Compounding the problem is the traditional practice of weighing high-school wrestlers only one hour before actual competition. Many young wrestlers try to make their weight class by sweating off pounds during the hours before the weighing-in. They vomit, pass water and don't drink any, and sweat until they've lost too much fluid. This is dangerous, because these youngsters will often take off as much as 9 to 13 percent of body weight during the twenty-four hours before weighing in. The resulting dehydration decreases strength, endurance, and cardiovascular function. And when weight is lost and rapidly regained, it comes back in the form of fat rather than protein, and actually leaves the young wrestler weaker than before.

Excessive weight loss is also fostered by the high-school wrestling system, which permits only one wrestler in each weight class. That means coaches must find a different weight category for each of their wrestlers, often through weight reduction. For example, if three wrestlers weigh 126 pounds, one must move down a category by losing 8 pounds while another moves up by gaining 10 pounds. A logical solution to this problem would be to permit *two* varsity competitors in each class. More young wrestlers could stay at their weight and there would be less pressure for excessive weight reduction.

◆   **What Parents Can Do**

Parents of young wrestlers should make sure that their children are not participating in weight-loss programs that may damage their health. Here are some guidelines for dealing with the problem:

Know the Regulations. All states have rules on the weight requirements of school wrestlers, and there are recommended national standards as well. Sources of information on these rules and standards are the team coach, the state association of wrestling coaches, the state athletic association, and the National Federation of State High-School Associations.

The following regulations are typical of those in most states:

1. Certified weight must be established before January 1.
2. There can be no change in weight certification after that date.
3. A growth of two pounds is allowed to January 1, one pound to February 1, and one more pound to March 1—for a total of four pounds in each weight class during the season. These allowances are for the natural growth of the young wrestler.
4. A one-pound gain is permitted after the first day of each successive competition during a meet.
5. A medical clearance is required for more than 5 percent loss of body weight.
6. A minimum intake of 1,200 calories per day is recommended, even when wrestlers are trying to lose weight.

If your school has its own written weight-requirement program, ask the wrestling coach for a copy.

Wisconsin's Weight Rules: Strictest Ever

The strictest state rule on how much weight a wrestler can lose and still compete was adopted by the Wisconsin Interscholastic Athletic Association (WIAA) in 1991. Many sports medical experts believe that the Wisconsin rule will become the basis for a national rule limiting wrestlers' weight loss.

According to the Wisconsin rule:

A wrestler's minimal weight will be at 7 percent fat, as predicted by the Lohman Equation, which is based on three skinfold measurements. There will be a 3 percent allowance on the Lohman Equation. Thus, if a wrestler's 7 percent predicted weight is 115 pounds, with the 3 percent allowance he will be able to wrestle at 112 pounds.

The predicted minimal weight must be on file in the WIAA office before the wrestler is involved in competition.

Track Your Son's Weight. Here's a good way to do this: Weigh your son on September 1 before school starts, and again on December 1, about two weeks before actual wrestling competition starts.

This three-month comparison will help you to determine if your young wrestler has adequately disciplined himself in meeting his weight goal. For example, if his weight on September 1 was 136 pounds and his objective is 126, you know that when he weighs 135 on December 1 that he hasn't done it right and is facing a crash diet. That could mean trouble. If he intends to lose more than 5 pounds after December 1 then a careful weight-loss study should be worked out together by the coach, the parent, and the physician.

Deal With Excessive Loss. Act promptly when you notice that your young wrestler is losing too much weight. Don't expect an easy time, because your son may strongly deny that the loss is excessive. You want to correct the problem, but at the same time you don't want to destroy your son's desire to wrestle or his self-discipline in achieving his goals.

Talk to his coach first. Ask the coach these questions:

- How much did your boy weigh before he started losing pounds and how much does the coach want him to lose?
- Is your boy's loss of weight allowable in terms of his percentage of body fat content? (The coach should know that according to the American Medical Association Sports Medical Committee, it's okay to lose 7 percent of body weight after four to six weeks of a weight-loss program.)
- Has your boy's weight loss been accomplished with wet suits, acute dehydration, restricted water, pills, or other improper weight-loss methods?

If you are uncomfortable with the coach's answers and still concerned about your son's weight loss, consult a sports physician who is knowledgeable about the standards of "making weight" in wrestling. You may have to do some looking, because few physicians know much about wrestling. However, there are some in every state, and if you live in a state with a strong wrestling program—such as Iowa, for example—chances are the school physician or team physician can answer your questions.

Wrestler's Weight Card

Good record-keeping is essential for tracking weight changes in a young wrestler. This form has been designed to make it easy for you to do this.

1. Name _____

2. School _____

3. Coach _____

4. Year _____

	1992	1993	1994	1995
September Weight				
September Body Fat %				
Weight Class Planned				
December Weight				
December Body Fat %				
Total Weight Loss				
Actual Weight Class				
January Weight				
Certified Weight				

Parent's Signature _____

◆ **WEIGHT LIFTING AND THE GROWING BODY**

Working with barbells, dumbbells, and weight-training machines to increase strength is now a widely used method for developing better athletes in many sports. Weight training can improve coordination, speed, and overall ability. These improvements not only lead to better performance but lessen the risk of injuries as well.

As a parent, you may have understandable concerns about weight lifting by your youngsters. You may envision them becoming muscle-bound incredible hulks. You may worry about the safety of "pumping iron." If your daughter is into weight lifting, you may fear she'll become muscular and unfeminine.

Fact: When done properly, weight lifting does not change young athletes' growth patterns—they will not grow faster or bigger than they would normally. Nor will they become muscle-bound—standard weight training actually improves muscle and joint flexibility.

Fact: Weight lifting is a safe activity when done properly. However, unsupervised or excessive lifting can lead to injuries that are sometimes serious. This makes it doubly important for parents to make sure that their youngsters are following approved methods for weight training and are not doing any unsupervised competitive weight lifting. Workout programs must be carefully laid out and monitored.

Fact: Many young women train with weights to keep their bodies firm and to improve athletic ability, and unless they overdo it, their feminine appearance is not affected.

Weight-lifting machines—such as those made by Nautilus, Universal, or Cybex—are becoming increasingly popular for weight training. However, it's necessary to join a fitness center to use these machines. Training with a set of free weights is far less expensive.

◆ Weight Lifting by Age Group

Here are some guidelines for dealing with weight lifting at various ages:

Eleven and Under. Some youth sports organizations sponsor weight-lifting programs for children as young as ten. Although lifting at such an early age provides some benefits, for most youngsters they are minimal in terms of increasing strength and competitive ability. When I see a very young lifter in my sports clinic, an aggressive father is usually pushing the child. I ask the father, "Where are you headed with this child?" Lifting is an excellent recreational activity with many benefits, but I would recommend it for children below twelve only when the youngster shows a positive interest in the activity—and at this age it must be carefully controlled and done on a low-key level.

Twelve and Thirteen. At these ages, the most important thing for you to know is whether the weight lifting is being properly supervised and the youngsters are not under pressure to lift excessive weights. Often, a group of kids will do their lifting in a neighbor's basement without supervision. That should be cause for alarm. It's a good idea to set up some rules and send them around to parents or youngsters in the group. And when a youngster at these ages is lifting at school, find out who is responsible for the program and how well it is planned and monitored.

Fourteen and Fifteen. Fourteen is a reasonable age to start a weight-training program—but only if the youngster is interested in lifting. Don't bring home a set of weights for your child and expect anything to happen. Let the drive and enthusiasm come from your athlete.

If your youngster is participating in a high-school lifting program at these ages, give your support but monitor what's going on. Learn something about weight training so you can ask your child intelligent questions: *How much are you pressing this week? How is the benching going? Are you over-lifting?*

Sixteen and Older. At these ages it's fine to encourage your youngsters to lift if they are inclined to sports competition. Let them know that weight training will enhance their agility, speed, and endurance and at the same time lessen chances of injury. You'll find that it also increases self-discipline and commitment to personal success.

In late adolescence, strength from weight training increases significantly, and for the first time the young weight lifter will be able to see changes in the mirror.

◆   Avoiding Weight-Lifting Injuries

Overuse weight-lifting injuries can occur to the back, the knee, and the shoulder. Back injuries can be prevented by not overlifting. Teenage lifters are not commonly troubled with knee injuries, but if they occur, care must be taken to prevent a chronic knee condition that could continue in later life. Shoulder injuries are more frequent in young lifters, but they are generally not serious and can be cared for easily.

Most injuries to young weight lifters happen at home because nobody is supervising. The worst injuries occur when the young athlete attempts to lift excessive weights and drops them. Though they can be serious, these injuries are rarely life threatening, frightening as they seem at the time.

The most important way to avoid weight-lifting injuries is to make sure lifting sessions are supervised by a coach or that the youngsters have a buddy system so that they never lift without a "spotter." Only light and medium lifting should be done at home. Another secret to preventing weight-lifting injuries is to coach youngsters in good technique before they start a program.

Keep in mind psychological factors as well. Except for some muscle strains and occasional tendinitis, teenage lifting is a very safe sport. The problem comes when one or two strong youngsters lift very heavy weights naturally, and other less powerful kids attempt to emulate them. This can be extremely dangerous, because a maximum effort with excessive weights sometimes causes "weight-lifter's blackout" when the lifter suddenly loses consciousness.

Checklist for Safe Weight Lifting

1. *Expert supervision*
2. *Proper equipment*
3. *Adequate lifting area*
4. *Clean lifting bars*
5. *Properly stored weights*
6. *Weights secured with clamps or bolts*
7. *Posted program plan*
8. *Spotters or buddy system*
9. *Written records of weights lifted, repetitions, etc.*
10. *Never lift alone*

Maximum lifting is not necessary for development and should not be done by teenagers. But since their competitive fervor is not likely to be restrained voluntarily, there's another good reason for supervising all heavy lifting by youngsters.

◆ **Guidelines for Weight-Lifting Programs**

Home Program

The safety rules specified in the preceding box are just as important for home lifting as for lifting in school programs. About half of weight-lifting injuries occur at home, so you must make sure your youngster adheres to these rules.

Unless you are knowledgeable about weight training, you won't know how much weight your youngster can safely lift. Your best bet is to ask your child's coach or a team coach for a written plan for your youngster's in-home lifting program. You might also learn some weight-lifting terminology, such as: *reps, curls, bench, flies*, and *max*. That can save you from appearing terminally stupid when you ask your youngster how the weight training is going.

The Basics of Weight Lifting

These guidelines can help you evaluate weight-lifting programs in which your youngster may be participating.

Frequency: *Lifting should not be done every day because muscle groups need time to recuperate. Three times a week is sufficient.*

Duration: *Thirty minutes per workout is recommended.*

Repetitions: *Five to six for heavy weights, ten to twelve for light.*

Sets: *Three sets per session per muscle group.*

Intensity: *Increase weights by 20 percent when ten reps are easy to perform.*

Timing: *Weight training should not be done during the playing season, because muscles are used differently in sports activities from the way they are in weight lifting.*

School Program

Most teenage weight lifting is done in high-school programs in areas specially set aside for lifting. The program may be supervised by a coach, a trainer, or occasionally a school parent. Whoever is in charge should have completed a course on weight training or be thoroughly knowledgeable about the subject. Always ask the weight-training supervisor for a written lifting program designed for your youngster (don't accept an oral explanation of the program because you will only be confused by all the technical terms involved). If your child also lifts at home, post this program in the lifting area.

Your most important question about the school lifting program should be: *Does it have adequate safeguards against overlifting?* Competitive youngsters tend to push themselves beyond safe limits, often under peer pressure from other young athletes. That's why you should make sure that:

- The program is supervised at all times.
- Maximum lifts (that is, the heaviest weight a youngster can possibly lift) are not allowed.
- The program is correctly adjusted to the sport—for example, baseball players don't need as heavy a lifting program as football players.
- Your youngster understands the principles of safe lifting.

Fitness Centers

At some point, your youngster may want to join a fitness center to work out on weight-training machines along with more advanced lifters. *Recommendation*: Before giving your permission, investigate the fitness center thoroughly. These centers vary widely in quality—some lack supervision and could be havens for steroid and other harmful drug use. Personally check out any center your young athlete is considering so that you know who the owner is, who is responsible for young lifters, and what safeguards are in place to prevent injury.

7

Nine Keys to Preventing Sports Injuries

◆

Ten-year-old Little League shortstop *Chris* suffered a fractured cheekbone when a sharply hit grounder took a bad hop and bounced into his face.

Fifteen-year-old high-school distance runner *Thelma* became weak and giddy while training in early September. It took immediate first-aid measures to help her recover quickly.

Sixteen-year-old football player *Kirk* suffered a severe separated shoulder when he tackled a charging ball-carrier.

Three different injuries, but all had something in common: *They could have been prevented.* If every safety practice and precaution recommended in this chapter were to be strictly followed in young people's sports, injuries like these would be reduced dramatically.

Let's look at them again:

Chris: Chris's league was playing with the traditional hard baseball. However, softer balls have been developed for the safety of younger players such as ten-year-old Chris. If this ball had been used by Chris's league, his injury would have been far less serious.

Thelma: Thelma was running on a hot, humid day and became ill from heat exhaustion. If the running-team trainer had measured the heat and humidity, he would have found a potentially lethal combination: 87 degrees and 96 percent humidity. The young athletes never should have been racing in these conditions.

Kirk: Kirk was wearing dangerously loose shoulder pads when he tackled the opposing runner. If they had been checked in the locker room before the game, he might not have suffered a separated shoulder.

There is no way to eliminate youth sports injuries completely, but these incidents show clearly that many injuries are caused by controllable factors. Their prevention depends on the actions and attitudes of everyone involved in youth sports, including administrators, coaches, trainers, physicians, and parents. Accidents can be minimized when all of these people coordinate their efforts to make sure that everything that can be done to prevent injuries *is* done.

Nine major elements must be considered in preventing youth sports injuries:

1. The Individual Athlete
2. Conditioning
3. Overuse Injuries
4. Coaching
5. Game Rules and Officials
6. Balanced Competition
7. Equipment
8. Athletic Facilities
9. Weather

◆ THE INDIVIDUAL ATHLETE

Some youngsters can be active in sports for years with no injuries, while others are constantly showing up in the sports-injury clinic. The most naturally gifted athletes tend to have the fewest injuries, because they move smoothly, see well, and are quick and well-balanced.

At the other extreme are the "injury prones"—young athletes who have repeated minor and major injuries. Although they may be capable athletes, these youngsters build up a thick record in the doctor's office.

In between these two groups are the vast majority of young athletes who suffer the injuries typical of their sport. Most of these injuries can be controlled and minimized by the recommendations in this chapter.

With injury-prone youngsters, however, the only solution may be for them to discontinue their sport. The first step is to find out why they are injured so often. They may not want to play in their particular sport. They may need better skills or they may simply not be sufficiently coordinated to compete in the sport. They may be physically immature, lack self-confidence, or have stressful family troubles. Any of these problems can lead to a high injury rate. Parents of these athletes should seek advice from a sports physician or other sports expert on whether their youngsters should continue their sport.

This can be a stressful situation, because the young athlete may not want to give up the sport (although some are grateful for a reprieve from constant aches and pains). Parents must be sure to give support and understanding to their youngster so that self-esteem is preserved. Above all, try to avoid expressing disappointment, frustration, or anger. Leaving a team should not be considered a failure, but a positive step.

◆   **Emotions and Injuries**

Some sports injuries result from emotional stress rather than physical factors. An upheaval at home or an apparent snub from a friend just before a game can lead to an injury brought on by loss of concentration. Being more emotionally fragile, young athletes are more likely than mature athletes to suffer injuries from mistakes in judgment or timing.

◆   **CONDITIONING**

Conditioning is the most important single key to injury prevention in young people's sports. Good conditioning tailored to a particular sport sharply reduces the likelihood of an injury.

What is conditioning? Basically, the process of preparing physically and mentally for participation in a given sport. Conditioning starts with developing motivation to compete and learning the sport and its rules. This is followed by physical exercising—getting into shape. Conditioning also includes developing good eating and sleeping habits.

Probably the most important factor in conditioning is timing. Conditioning must begin *well before a season starts*. Otherwise, the young athlete will start competition too soon and be vulnerable to injury. Be sure to give support to your youngster's conditioning program—know what it involves, listen to complaints, and provide encouragement. Make sure your youngster understands the importance of conditioning as a way of preventing injuries. Be your youngster's personal cheerleader.

Although specific conditioning techniques vary from sport to sport, five key components apply to most sports:

1. Endurance
2. Strength
3. Flexibility
4. Speed
5. Skill

Progressive training in all five aspects is essential for good conditioning.

◆ Endurance

A top-priority element, endurance means being able to play a sport without getting out of breath or letting up too soon. The heart and lungs should be working with the muscles to permit constant movement without fatigue. If you see any signs that your youngster lacks this endurance, poor conditioning may be the culprit.

Endurance is best developed by a well-planned running schedule and/or by steady, forceful exercise such as swimming, biking, or rope jumping. There are many well-established programs for developing good endurance. Ask your youngster's coach for a copy of the program he or she uses.

◆ Strength

Strength conditioning is not important until the teenage years (although weight lifting by preteens is on the increase). When the adult hormones begin to function around age fourteen, both males and females can significantly increase their strength through weight lifting or other forms of exercise. As was pointed out in the previous chapter, the stronger young athletes become, the less likely they are to be injured.

Many youngsters inherit their strength or develop it through good nutrition and good health. They are stronger to start with and will get even stronger from weight lifting.

◆ Flexibility

Muscles, tendons, and joints are more susceptible to injury if they are not sufficiently flexible before competition. Flexibility is achieved by stretching, which takes two forms: 1) preseason stretching that begins weeks before actual competition, and 2) stretching done immediately before competition or practice. Both types are essential.

Preseason stretching should be moderate at first, gradually increasing to the point where maximum flexiblity is achieved without excess force or pain. With youngsters, this should take a few weeks.

Precompetition stretching will vary by the sport and the individual athlete.

Some young bodies are not built to stretch very far, making them susceptible to overstretching injuries. Parents should make sure that the preseason physical includes flexiblity tests, so that a special stretching program can be designed for the "tight" youngster. At the other extreme are hyperelastic youngsters with very loose joints, who should also avoid overstretching. Inquire about the flexibility program planned for your youngster—the coach should be able to supply you with a set of written instructions.

One warning about stretching: Overstretching is common in high-school sports and can cause serious problems. Many so-called hamstring injuries are actually back and sciatic nerve injuries from excessive stretching.

◆ Speed

Most fast young athletes have "gene" speed, a natural gift they're born with. However, slower youngsters can improve their speed with a well-supervised speed-training program.

◆ Skill

Regardless of a young athlete's natural ability, every sport has specific skills that must be learned. Of all five major conditioning components, skill is most directly related to avoiding injuries. Whether natural or acquired, sport skills provide the agility needed for safe performance. Examples: turning a lacrosse stick to catch the ball without hitting a teammate, turning your shoulder to avoid a hit in hockey, and handling a soccer ball to avoid a collision.

◆ Conditioning in Youth-League Sports

Many youth-league programs lack well-defined conditioning plans. Don't be overly concerned, because preteen youngsters don't really need (or appreciate) the rigorous physical conditioning they require in later years. Their metabolism is so high, they will run and fall forever without hurting themselves. It is important, however, for them to warm up before practice or a game. These warmups should be made as relaxed and enjoyable as possible—for example, by having short races or a game of tag.

For these preteen youngsters, the most important conditioning is what I call "value conditioning." This means learning some useful principles to guide them in their youth-league activity, such as the meaning of teamwork and that having fun is more important than winning or losing.

◆ Conditioning in High-School Sports

For the teenager, conditioning should start long before the season gets under way. For fall sports, it should start in early August; for winter sports, in September; and for spring sports, in January.

Most state athletic associations prohibit formal practice until one to three weeks before the season, so it is up to the youngsters themselves to start getting into shape earlier. In major high-school sports such as football, soccer, and field hockey, informal conditioning often starts with *captain's practices* held weeks before the regular conditioning season. To preserve equality of competition, state rules usually forbid the team coach from attending these training sessions. However, to prevent injuries and manage the conditioning program, parental supervision is recommended.

Making Warm-Ups Fun

For youngsters in league sports, warm-ups should be made as enjoyable as possible. Here's a suggested program:

- *Jumping jacks, running in place (1 minute)*
- *Stretching, touching toes, standing and sitting with legs apart, swinging arms (1 minute)*
- *Running around the field (3 minutes)*
- *Playing tag, running short races, etc. (5 minutes)*
- *Doing sport-specific warm-ups; kicking ball, throwing, etc. (times can vary)*
- *Training youngsters in specific skills such as ball control (times can vary)*

Early-Season Injuries

Care must be taken at the beginning of the actual season to avoid injuries from insufficient conditioning. In contact sports, the highest percentage of injuries occur during the first weeks of the season, while fewer occur toward the end, when the players are in top condition.

Unfortunately, some coaches striving for a championship season aggressively push their players early in the season before they are properly conditioned. This not only harms the players but is self-defeating, because these coaches often lose their best athletes to injuries.

◆   Conditioning in Individual Sports

Because they perform their sports throughout the year, most young individual sports athletes are always in good condition. These include gymnasts, swimmers, skaters, fencers, tennis players, and those involved in martial arts. But to be on the safe side, parents should monitor the condition of these youngsters.

If individual competitors do lay off for some weeks, they should return to their training level gradually under the supervision of their coach. An intense push for one particular event can mean an injury that could set the youngster back for some time.

◆   OVERUSE INJURIES

Cindy, a sixteen-year-old distance runner, was second in her state championships last year. She was intent on winning all her meets as captain of the running team but was forced to delay training in the summer because of a virus infection. She began running hard in late August. Just two days before her first meet, her left leg became severely painful about three inches below the knee. Early X rays

Overuse Injuries in Children

These are the most common overuse injuries suffered by young athletes.

Upper Extremity:
- *Swimmer's shoulder*
- *Little League elbow*

Back:
- *Back strain*
- *Back strain with sciatica*
- *Stress fracture (spondylolisthesis)*

Lower Extremity:
- *Stress fractures*
- *Kneecap (patella) stress*
- *Osgood-Schlatter's condition (knee)*
- *Jumper's knee*
- *Osteochondritis dissecans (knee)*
- *Shin splints*
- *Soccer toe*
- *Sever's condition (heel)*

were negative, but a bone scan showed that she had a stress fracture of her leg.

Eighteen-year-old *George* has been an outstanding basketball player since the eighth grade. He played in the summer league and shot "hoops" all fall. By October, his knees were hurting most of the time. When the pain didn't let up even after several days' rest, he went to the local sports clinic, where he was diagnosed as having "jumper's knee."

Now thirteen, *Kevin* has been pitching in Little League baseball since he was nine. Last year he had some arm soreness, but he didn't stop pitching. In winter practice, the arm still bothered him. This spring, while he was throwing hard in the second game of the season, the pain got so bad he had to leave the game. After four weeks of rest, his arm still hurt. His condition was diagnosed as "Little League elbow," and the doctor recommended that he stop pitching for a whole year and play another position instead.

These are three typical overuse injuries—sometimes called stress injuries. They occur when too much stress is put on a specific part of the body involved in an athletic activity. Although these particular overuse injuries occurred to teenagers, this type of injury is showing up more and more in very young children, especially those active in as many as four sports at one time.

There are two basic kinds of overuse injuries in sports. One occurs at the beginning of the season before the athlete is fully conditioned for actual competition. The other can occur at any time in certain sports where the same physical motion is used repeatedly—for example, swimming, gymnastics, and basketball. These injuries can happen in any extended-use sport that involves stretching, excessive throwing, or forceful running.

Not all overuse injuries are preventable, because it's impossible to predict how hard any individual athlete can perform. But most overuse injuries *can* be prevented through proper conditioning and training. Here are some guidelines for specific sports that your youngster can use to help prevent overuse injuries.

TRACK & CROSS-COUNTRY
Injuries:
Overuse injuries are very common in these sports. They include shin splints, stress fractures, kneecap stress, road-runner's knee, and back strain with *sciatica*.
Prevention:
1. Run early in the summer. Increase distance gradually, but don't increase distance and speed together. Your coach will probably give you a running plan; if not, develop one yourself well before the season starts and submit it to the coach for review.
2. Prepare for the intensive program the coach will use in double sessions, involving hours of conditioning and training twice a day.
3. If you have to start double sessions without adequate

preparation, run only 50 percent of the program and move up very slowly.

4. Do very easy stretching for the first two weeks of the season and keep stretching during the season.

FIELD HOCKEY

Injuries:

A fall sport with frequent overuse complaints such as hamstring pulls, shin splints, stress fractures, knee pain, and backaches.

Prevention:

1. Stretch early and gradually for first two weeks.
2. Start a gradual running program in early August.
3. Do agility exercises for back flexibility.

SOCCER

Injuries:

Shin splints, tendinitis of the ankle, foot, and toe. Occasional stress fractures and back strain.

Prevention:

1. Stretch early and gradually for first two weeks.
2. Start an early, gradual running program.
3. Do agility exercises for back flexibility.
4. Start ball handling and kicking six weeks before the season.

FOOTBALL

Injuries:

Stress injuries are common, along with hamstring pulls and back strains.

Prevention:

1. Start progressive weight training in June.
2. Start running program in July.
3. Start stretching exercises in early August.

BASKETBALL

Injuries:

The most common overuse injury is "jumper's knee," which is tendinitis below the kneecap. Other frequent injuries are back strains and foot sprains. Stress fractures are uncommon.

Prevention:

1. Start running program in July.
2. If older than fourteen, start weight-lifting program in August.
3. To relieve jumper's knee, rest between basketball games.

ICE HOCKEY

Injuries:

Groin pulls, backaches, shoulder sprains.

Prevention:

1. Stretching exercises.
2. If older than fourteen, lift weights.
3. Start progressive ice drills.

BASEBALL

Injuries:

Little League elbow (tendinitis) and rotator cuff tendinitis in the shoulder.

Prevention:

1. Thorough training in pitching.
2. Gradual conditioning of the arm by early preseason throwing.
3. Weight-training and stretching program for pitchers over thirteen.

SWIMMING

Injuries:

Shoulder tendinitis, knee strain.

Prevention:

1. Early stretching program.
2. Do moderate times and distances in early training sessions.
3. Weight-training program for the older youth.
4. Do proper amount of training during the season.

GYMNASTICS

Injuries:

Back strains, stress fractures, and wrist tendinitis.

Prevention:
Prevention is difficult, but progressive stretching can help.

These are the sports in which overuse injuries most commonly occur. However, athletes can suffer stress injuries in any sport where the training or competition is intensive and repetitive. To read more about specific sports injuries caused by overuse, see Part IV: *Home Reference Guide to Sports Injuries.*

◆   **COACHING**

Coaches play a key role in preventing young people's sports injuries. They do this by:

- Instilling discipline, a critical element in injury prevention
- Effectively conditioning their young athletes
- Teaching the rules of the game, many of which are designed to prevent injuries
- Teaching the skills and techniques of the sport
- Demanding good sports conduct during competition
- Making sure that every safety precaution has been taken and that an effective program is in place to care for injuries

A high-school coach's role is very different from that of a college or professional coach. The latter two can recruit or draft their players, while high-school coaches must work with whatever youngsters attend the school, whether they're big and strong or small and weak. So high-school coaches need even more sensitivity to the problems of injury prevention.

That doesn't mean that a coach shouldn't demand hard play and perseverance from everyone on the team. A team should play to win. But the goal of winning should be balanced against equally important goals: injury prevention, full participation, and character development.

Because coaches are so important in preventing injuries, parents should make an effort to understand coaching and what makes a good coach. They should also get to know the coach who is supervising their youngster and try to establish a good rapport. Most coaches care about the youngsters under their guidance and understand the importance of preventing injuries. And when an athlete does get injured, I have seen coaches sit in emergency rooms or my office for hours, missing meals and family events, to be sure a young boy or girl receives proper treatment.

◆   How to Rate a Coach

As with any professional group, not all coaches meet the standards for good coaching. That's why you should carefully evaluate the ability and character of any coach in charge of your youngster's athletic activities. Here's what to look for:

Leadership

Coaches should be role models who project healthy sports values to their young charges. Good coaches encourage each player; instill discipline, self-reliance, and confidence; keep their word; and refrain from abuse and threats.

Giving Priority to Injury Prevention

The win-at-all-costs syndrome is responsible for many unnecessary injuries. A track coach may push tired runners to go on when they are obviously unfit to continue. A football coach may keep a player with a minor injury in the game despite the risk that it will turn into a major injury.

On the other hand, a good coach puts care of the player first, even in the frenzy of a crucial game. It's not easy when the coach is under pressure to produce a victory. But I've known a football coach who, whenever I recommended that one of his best players be taken out of the game, told me, "Just take good care of him." That's the kind of coach you should be looking for.

Going by the Rules

Although game officials enforce the rules during competition, coaches are responsible for teaching them and insisting that they be followed. Too often, injuries result from flagrant violations of rules that were designed to keep a sport safe. A prime example is high-school ice hockey, where numerous injuries occur from late hits, high sticking, and other abusive play. Coaches must severely discipline any team member guilty of such behavior.

Teaching Skills

Teaching the fundamental skills of a sport helps a team to win, of course. But it also helps to prevent injuries. For example, a properly executed football block is less likely to result in injury than a poorly executed block. In baseball, a pitcher with good ball control will seldom injure a batter. Good stick control in ice hockey, field hockey, and lacrosse is essential to avoid injury. It should be the coach's responsibility to teach these skills—and to keep players off the field until they've learned them.

Providing First Aid

A coach should be well-trained in basic first aid and have an organized plan for dealing with emergencies. Has the coach completed a course in CPR (cardiopulmonary resuscitation)?

Meeting Professional Standards

Some states require formal certification for high-school and youth-league coaches (check with your state athletic association or youth league to find out if your state is one). All coaches should meet a set of professional standards by passing a comprehensive educational program.

◆   Working With the Coach

A good relationship with the coach can make it much easier for you when safety questions come up or your youngster is injured. Most coaches will welcome input from a parent so long as the parent reciprocates by trying to understand the reasoning behind the coach's decisions, rules, and policies. So before getting up in arms about a coach's actions find out why the coach took them. Keep in mind that an excellent coach should not make exceptions from the rules simply because an athlete is outstanding.

Recommendation: Spend time with the coach and talk frankly about your concerns. If you belong to a boosters club of school parents, ask the coach to attend a meeting. Listen to the coach's explanations of his or her program and support it if it seems sound. (These measures establish a solid basis for good "injury interaction," which we'll discuss in Chapter 11.)

◆   GAME RULES AND OFFICIALS

It's Friday-night high-school football. Three minutes into the first quarter, an Eagle linebacker deliberately spears a Falcon ball carrier. Without hesitation, the referee blows his whistle, penalizes the Eagles fifteen yards, and warns both coaches that such dangerous play will not be tolerated. There is no spearing for the rest of the game.

A youth-league hockey game is filled with high sticking, hitting from behind, and fights. No attempt is made by the game officials to control the violence. When the game ends, a bench-clearing brawl results in several injuries.

Just before a championship track meet is to begin, officials check the pole-vault facilities. After finding a broken vaulting box and inadequate landing pads, they cancel the pole-vault event.

Every sport has carefully thought-out rules—many of them created to prevent unnecessary injuries. But, like any rules, sports rules are only as good as their enforcement. That's up to the game officials: referees, umpires, and judges. They have a major responsibility for preventing injuries during a competitive event. The tone they set at the beginning of the event and the consistency with which they make their "calls" are keys to protecting the young athletes.

Because of their important safety role, game officials should only be qualified adults. Qualifications should include passing written and practical examinations and gaining first-hand experience under supervision.

Most game officials carry out their responsibilities well. However, a small percentage have a problem curbing violent play. Obviously, you should be concerned about officials who are lax about enforcing rules designed to prevent injuries.

◆   What Parents Can Do

Here are some guidelines for making sure that any competitive event in which your youngster participates is well officiated:

1. Get a copy of the rules for your youngster's sport and learn them. This won't entitle you to become a referee, but it will arm you with the information you need to know if safety rules are being enforced.
2. Discuss the rules with your youngster, especially those that relate to safety. Let your youngster know that you take these rules seriously, and that he/she should too.
3. Learn enough about game officiating to be able to tell the good from the bad.
4. Never abuse a game official from the stands during competition. Sure your kid was safe at home—is that umpire blind or something? But far too many parents think that a "bad call" gives them free license to heap verbal—often profane—abuse on the offending official. Besides being unfair, this sets a poor example for your children and distracts officials from carrying out their responsibilities, one of which is to prevent injuries. Of course, officials make bad calls occasionally—don't we all? This doesn't mean you

should never complain to a game official. Just do it privately and quietly after the game—and focus on any lax enforcement of the rules that took place.

5. After a game, also ask your youngster if the official made it clear from the start that the rules would be rigidly enforced and that excessive brutality, dangerous plays, and unsportsmanlike conduct would not be tolerated.

6. If you felt that the officiating of a game was not acceptable, let your youngster's coach know, preferably in writing.

◆ **BALANCED COMPETITION**

Rick and *Don* play for their respective high-school football teams, which are traditional archrivals. They are both fifteen years old, but there the resemblance ends. Rick is 5'11" and weighs a muscular 185 pounds. Don is 5'3" and weighs an undeveloped 95 pounds. When they collide in a game, guess who's going to get hurt.

Such imbalance is the exception rather than the rule, but it does happen. And it occurs when teams are matched according to chronological age rather than developmental age. With a serious imbalance of physical size, strength, and maturity, injuries are inevitable—sometimes severe injuries. The danger is not only from sheer physical differences but from bigger players who lack the emotional maturity to go along with their physical development and don't restrain themselves in the excitement of play.

It's important to keep competition balanced with youngsters of similar size and skills—particularly with young male athletes between fourteen and eighteen. This concern is not so great for young female athletes, since they are not involved in such power sports as football and wrestling.

Several systems have been developed to help schools and sports organizations equalize youth competition by size and physical maturity. One of them is the *Tanner Staging System*, developed by a British physician. If there is a question about your youngster's ability to play with others of the same age, you might ask your pediatrician about this system. However, being rather cumbersome, it is not widely used.

In most cases, the decision must be left up to the common sense of those who are putting teams together, including the physician doing the preparticipation physical. It usually doesn't take an expert to figure out that a youngster doesn't belong on a team, whether because of comparative underdevelopment or overdevelopment. Nor is it difficult to see when two teams scheduled to play each other are badly mismatched physically. In this case, the coach of the dominating team should use second-string players instead of the varsity.

What if you're the parent of a mismatched youngster? It's not an easy situation to resolve, but keep these suggestions in mind:

- Be willing to accept the fact that your youngster should not be on the team. It's easy to let ego get in the way—after all, you want to feel that your child is as capable as others the same age. But your primary concern should be the safety and well-being of your youngster.
- Help your youngster cope with the disappointment of being put off the team. This can be a devastating blow to self-esteem, and your youngster needs your support and understanding.

◆   EQUIPMENT

Dennis didn't think he needed his headgear for wrestling practice because he was only working out with the junior varsity. After two practice matches, he developed a severe swelling over his right ear caused by bleeding. It took extensive treatment and three weeks for the injury to heal, and to this day Dennis has a "cauliflower" ear.

Eileen forgot to take her protective sport glasses to a school tennis match. While playing doubles, she was struck in the eye by a hard-hit ball and was hospitalized for twenty-four hours under observation to make sure the eye was not seriously injured.

Helen didn't wear her mouth guard during a field hockey match. During the game, she was hit hard in the mouth by another player's stick and lost two teeth.

These three cases illustrate an important point to keep in mind about preventing sports injuries to your youngsters: *Most kids are not concerned about safety.* They consider themselves indestructible. When their helmet is loose, their face mask is broken, or their shoes are too big, chances are they'll ignore these potential invitations to injury. That's why it's up to you to make sure they wear proper equipment in good condition.

Your first step is to learn as much as you can about the specific equipment required in your youngster's sport (either by attending a sports medical night for parents or by asking the coach). Armed with this knowledge, you can ask intelligent questions of your youngster, such as: *Does your helmet fit without wobbling or can you turn it around on your head even when the chin strap is buckled? Is the chin strap tight and in good condition? Do you always tighten the screws on your face mask? Are you running six miles in cross-country in the same sneakers you wear every day to school? Are your shin guards snug?* These questions let your youngster know that you have a sincere interest in his or her injury prevention.

If your youngster is in *youth-league sports* or *individual sports*, you are responsible for purchasing the necessary equipment. For guidance on buying the best, consult your youngster's coach and other parents, or ask the athletic director in your local high school. After purchasing the equipment, make sure your youngster knows how to use it properly. Periodically check the equipment for wear and tear so you will know when to replace it.

In *school sports*, the athletic director purchases the equipment, while the coaches and trainers are responsible for making sure it is properly fitted and maintained. It generally won't be new, but the school should clean and recondition it annually. In addition to making sure the equipment is in good condition, you should see that it fits properly.

Here's what you should know about various types of equipment.

◆ Personal Equipment

Personal equipment is equipment that your youngster will be keeping at home. Try to instill a sense of discipline about keeping this equipment clean, well-stored, and in good condition.

SPORT GLASSES

Sport glasses can be expensive, but they absolutely should be worn in any sport were the eyes are at risk, such as tennis. Sport glasses are made of impact-resistant frames with polycarbonate lenses. Ideally, your youngster should have two pairs.

MOUTH GUARD

The mouth guard is now required safety equipment in all contact/collision sports and most limited contact/impact sports. Since it was introduced in the 1950s, it has almost eliminated loss of teeth and sharply reduced mouth and facial injuries.

Your youngster should have a properly fitting mouth guard and use it for all practice and competition. It can be either a standard model fitted by the trainer or coach, or a custom model molded by your youngster's dentist. Make sure it is large enough to cover your youngster's teeth.

UNDERWEAR

Sports underwear *must be clean*. I have seen a whole football team laid low by a staph infection for an entire season because of unsanitary clothing worn by one youngster.

BRAS

Sports bras prevent overstretching of the ligaments that support the breasts and limit excessive breast motion.

STOCKINGS

Cleanliness is essential. Infections and athlete's foot can eliminate a player for days. Also, stockings folded up at the toes can cause blisters.

SHOES

Well-fitted shoes are essential. Shoes that are tight, loose, not broken in, or have broken shoe laces can cause serious blisters. A good rule of thumb (literally) is that if there is one-half inch between the two laced edges and a thumb can be placed beyond the tip of the big toe, the shoe fits well and should be comfortable.

JOCKSTRAPS

These are essential for all developed young male athletes. They must be clean and well-fitted.

PROTECTIVE CUPS

Should be added to the jockstrap for baseball catchers and hockey goalies.

PELVIC PROTECTOR

Should be worn by female goalies playing contact/collision or limited contact/impact sports.

◆   Game Equipment

Sports safety equipment has been tremendously improved over the past twenty-five years.

HELMETS

This is the most important protective equipment in football, hockey, lacrosse, cycling, baseball, wrestling,

---

Fitting a Helmet

A helmet will not provide good protection unless it fits. Here are five tips on getting a proper fit:
1. *It should be snug when in place.*
2. *There should be only one to two inches between the eyebrows and the ridge of the helmet.*
3. *With the chin strap in place, there should be no motion when the face mask is pulled down or twisted.*
4. *The chin strap should be tight, centered, and always kept snapped.*
5. *Jaw pads must be fitted and snug against the face.*

---

equestrian sports, and boxing. But helmets won't do their job unless they are properly fitted (see box). And they must be in good condition—helmets that have been passed on from year to year can be loose, soft, cracked, and have stretched insets that make proper fit impossible.

FACE MASKS

Protective face masks are required for all participants in football, hockey, lacrosse, fencing, and for baseball and softball catchers. Since masks have been required in these sports, injuries about the face and head have been greatly reduced. They are also recommended for all youth-league baseball players while at bat (see page 19).

SHOULDER PADS

These are important in football, hockey, and lacrosse, providing protection against collarbone fractures, stingers, separated shoulders, and neck injuries. To give this protection, the pads must fit well and be in good repair.

ELBOW PADS

Used in hockey and wrestling, these pads should be well-fitted.

RIB PADS

These pads are worn in football, hockey, and lacrosse to protect against rib injuries. The best pads are expensive, so a team trainer will often simply use soft padding.

THIGH PADS

Also used in football, hockey, and lacrosse, these pads can help to prevent serious thigh injuries. Fitting is important: The pads should not slide and should not be too high or too low.

KNEE GUARDS AND PADS

These are soft, elastic, padded supports designed to protect the knee from skin abrasions, bruises, and sprains. They are used in football, hockey, lacrosse, basketball, and volleyball.

PREVENTIVE KNEE BRACES

Several knee braces have been developed to protect the normal knee from being injured in football. However, there is still insufficient evidence that they are of any value. Because of this, and their expense, most teams don't purchase them. Parents should feel free to buy them if they wish.

THERAPEUTIC KNEE BRACES

These braces are used to protect injured knees in any sport that requires running and pivoting.

SHIN GUARDS

An absolute necessity for all players in soccer and field hockey, for catchers in baseball and softball, and for goalies in all sports.

GLOVES

Two types of gloves are used in sports: functional gloves (baseball) and protective gloves (lacrosse, hockey). They should be made of quality materials and properly fitted.

ICE SKATES

Skates should be properly fitted and the blades must be kept sharp. It's okay to wear skates without socks.

TRACK SHOES

These should fit well, with spikes of the regulation number and length, well screwed into the sole.

STICKS

Sticks are used in ice hockey, field hockey, and lacrosse. Each sport has its specific regulations on length, shape, weight, curves, pockets, etc.

BASEBALL BATS

Bats should meet the prescribed standards for weight, size, and construction.

BASEBALLS

The most serious injuries in baseball are from being hit with a pitched or batted ball traveling at high speed—between 1973 and 1983, thirty-five youngsters died from such accidents. In an innovative response to this problem, one leading baseball maker, Worth Sports Company (Tullahoma, Tenn.) developed a "soft" baseball in 1985 that it claims performs as well as the traditional hard ball when used in Little League play. A similar product is the INCREDIBALL, made by Easton Sports (Burlingame, Calif.). This new type of ball has been approved by the Little League, although it's meeting with some sales resistance because it doesn't make the same sharp sound that the hard ball does when hit by a bat.

Quick Guide to Equipment Safety

Equipment can effectively help to reduce injuries if these guidelines are followed:
1. *Don't practice or play without the proper equipment.*
2. *Make sure the equipment fits well at all times.*
3. *Don't use broken equipment.*
4. *Keep the equipment clean.*
5. *Don't alter any equipment without permission.*

BASEBALL MASKS

Although baseball catchers always wear protective masks behind the plate, batters normally wear only helmets. To prevent injuries to teeth, jawbones, eyes, and noses, Home Safe Face Guards Company (Roanoke, Va.) sells a clear plastic shield that attaches to the sides of a standard batting helmet and covers the chin to the tip of the nose. The eyes, though exposed, are protected from direct contact by the top of the guard and the rim of the helmet. Another type of face mask, made of welded wire, is sold by Schutt Manufacturing (Litchfield, Ill.) Both types of masks not only prevent facial injuries but help to reduce the fear of being at the plate.

◆ ATHLETIC FACILITIES

A sports facility should be safe for your young athlete, whether it's a field, a court, a rink, or a track. Although specific safety requirements vary from sport to sport, one basic rule applies to all: *Before any practice session or competitive event, the facility must be carefully inspected and all obstructions and hazards must be removed.*

◆ Facilities in Youth-League Sports

A variety of facilities are used by youth leagues: the school gym for basketball, recreational parks for many sports, private and publicly owned rinks for hockey, private and public gymnasiums, school tracks, and private and public swimming pools. Parents cannot personally check these facilities, but should know who is responsibile for maintaining them. If you have concerns about the safety of the facility—for example, the condition of the ice before a hockey game—talk to the person responsible.

◆ Facilities in Individual Sports

Take the same precautions for facilities in individual sports as you do for those in youth-league sports. Generally speaking, coaches of individual sports are very safety conscious.

◆ Facilities in School Sports

In high-school sports, the athletic director is responsible for maintaining facilities. But at the time of competition, the team coach decides whether the facilities are safe. The responsible coach will cancel or forfeit a game rather than use facilities that don't meet safety standards.

Safe facilities cost money, which is in short supply for most high schools. Parents can do their part by helping to make repairs themselves or contributing money through cake sales, raffles, and other fund-raising activities.

◆ Guidelines for Safe Sports Facilities

Here are some of the more important safety requirements for various types of athletic facilities:

Grass Playing Fields (*football, soccer, field hockey, lacrosse, rugby, etc.*)

- Uniform surface free of ruts and grooves
- No obstructions on the sidelines, such as wooden or metal stakes
- Benches and equipment placed so that players will not run into them
- All playing lines clearly marked with a safe chemical (not lime)
- Padded goalposts, flexible flags, and rubberized sideline markers

Baseball/Softball Diamonds

- Smooth surface
- Firmly attached bases with a breakaway mechanism
- Smooth home plate
- Flat, stable pitcher's rubber
- Outfield and infield free of potholes and clear of hazardous obstructions
- Secure fences free of projections and obstructions

Track and Field Facilities

- Clear of all obstructions and equipment
- Outdoor track: smooth surface with well-marked lanes
- Indoor track: clear infield area at edge of track, surface in good repair, track well-secured if portable, wall padding for sprints
- Well-balanced hurdles in good condition
- Properly placed high-jump landing pad in good condition
- Properly sanded long-jump and triple-jump pit and lane with secure take-off board
- For pole vaults, safe, well-placed landing pad, secure vaulting box, and poles in good condition
- Open, clear fields for javelin, discus, and shot put

Ice Rinks

- Clear, properly swept ice surface free from cracks and ruts
- Boards in good repair and clear of projecting objects

- Closed gates with clear frames that are firm, fixed, and nonbreakable
- Movable nets

Indoor Playing Courts (*basketball, volleyball, racquetball, etc.*)

- Dry, nonslippery surface kept clean during games
- Clear area behind basket
- Spectators at a safe distance from court

Outdoor Playing Courts (*tennis, volleyball, etc.*)

- Clean, well-marked surface
- Unobstructed sidelines

Gymnastics Facilities

- Well-built equipment, firmly secured and balanced
- Each unit tested before every practice and event
- Well-placed, secure dismounting pads of proper thickness

Wrestling Facilities

- Clean mats in good repair, with a sufficient apron

Swimming Pools

- Properly maintained chlorine and pH levels
- Clear apron
- Adequate depth for safe entry and for diving competition

◆   WEATHER

They can't control the weather, but coaches, game officials, and parents *can* control the sports activities of their young athletes in dangerous weather conditions. The greatest danger is from extreme heat. Extreme cold and lightning are also major hazards.

◆ Heat

Death from heat stroke in young people's sports is rare, but it can happen and it's preventable. Consider this a grave hazard and take steps to make sure it doesn't happen to your youngster. Learn the specific dangers of practicing or playing in high heat and humidity, what preventive measures to take, and the proper treatment when an emergency does occur. Warn your youngster about heat exhaustion and heat stroke, and make sure that those supervising your youngster's athletic activities have a program in place to prevent heat illness and deal with it if it occurs.

Heat problems are most likely during intensive football practice sessions in late August and early September. Although most coaches and certified trainers are aware of the hazard, student trainers and teachers doubling as trainers may not be.

Young track runners can also suffer heat illness, but it's less likely than in football players.

Measuring Heat and Humidity

Heat illness becomes a potential problem when the temperature exceeds 85 F and the humidity is more than 70 percent. At this point, the coach and trainer should be looking for trouble, watching for abnormal movements or bizarre actions of the players that could indicate heat illness. If that happens, adjustments should be made in the practice schedule. In some severe conditions, practice should be suspended.

Treating Heat Illness

Three types of heat illness can affect young athletes:
Cramps. The least serious, cramps are a temporary problem caused by loss of fluid and salt in the muscles. The cramps can be eliminated easily by drinking water and resting.
Heat Exhaustion. This is a more serious consequence of water and salt loss, caused by excessive sweating. It is reversible but dangerous, and should be treated immediately.

What to Look For

- Cool, clammy skin
- Pallor
- Weakness or fatigue
- Sweating
- Nausea
- Normal temperature
- Giddiness
- Rapid heartbeat

Immediate Field Treatment

- Move athlete to shady area to rest
- Provide plenty of cool water to drink
- Apply water—wet towels, etc.—to body
- Elevate legs
- Don't take chances, send athlete to hospital

Heat Stroke. The most dangerous heat illness, caused by overheating of the body from inability to sweat. *Heat stroke is a major emergency that can be fatal or cause permanent brain damage.*

What to Look For

- Hot, dry skin
- Flushed face
- Confusion or coma
- *No* sweating
- High body temperature: 104–108 F
- Headache
- Rapid heartbeat

Immediate Field Treatment

- Call ambulance right away
- Undress athlete in shade
- Sponge or hose ice-cold water over entire body

- Administer intravenous fluids, if available from emergency medical technician
- Send patient to hospital as soon as ambulance arrives

Keys to Preventing Heat Illness

Parents should make sure that coaches and trainers are following these recommended procedures for preventing heat illness during practice sessions in hot, humid weather.

1. When the weather is a threat, cancel practice sessions or make adjustments in the day's program. (Keep the telephone number for weather information handy.)
2. Identify athletes susceptible to heat illness—those who have had a sharp loss of weight or a history of recent illness or head injuries are particularly vulnerable.
3. Schedule practice sessions in early morning and evening.
4. Require loose white clothing: short-sleeve shirts with tails out. If practice is noncontact, lightweight pants or shorts can be worn.
5. Don't allow helmets to be worn except during contact drills.
6. Reduce exercises and running to a slow pace.
7. Provide plenty of rest in the shade between sessions.
8. Make water available at all times and see that it's consumed.
9. Be alert for abnormal movements or bizarre actions by the athletes.
10. Weigh players at the beginning and end of each day's practice, and carefully observe those losing excess daily weight.

◆ Cold

Extreme cold can create two problems for young athletes: *frostbite* and *hypothermia*. Both are potentially serious and require emergency attention. Preventive measures should be taken in all winter sports, such as downhill skiing, cross-country skiing, and cold-weather mountaineering. Summer and fall mountaineering can also be dangerous because of rapid weather changes at high altitudes. Exposure to cold ocean water is another hazard.

Frostbite

Frostbite is caused by loss of circulation in the fingers, toes, ears, or nose from exposure to below-freezing temperatures. The toes are most frequently affected, and in extreme cases the entire foot could be lost.

What to Look For

- Pain in toes, fingers, nose, or ears (not always present)
- Tingling, numbness, and a leathery feeling to the touch
- Fingers or toes appear bluish or waxy white

Immediate Treatment

- Remove gloves or socks
- Thaw affected parts carefully so as not to burn
- Obtain medical assistance as soon as possible

Prevention

- Know the weather conditions where your youngster is going
- Provide warm clothing for the entire body as well as hands and feet
- Avoid tight shoes, gloves, lacing, or bindings

Hypothermia

Hypothermia is the loss of body temperature from exposure to the cold. Inadequate clothing and dehydration are usually responsible. As the body cools, it loses its vitality; its strength; and, eventually, its ability to survive.

Normal temperature is 98.6 F. A temperature of 90 to 97 F indicates mild to moderate hypothermia, while temperatures below 90 F indicate severe hypothermia—a major medical emergency with danger of death. In the mountains, prevention and early recognition are critical because nearby medical help is usually not available.

What to Look For

- Shivering
- Slowness of pace
- Lethargy, inattentiveness, withdrawal
- Inability to perform simple tasks like buttoning shirt
- Slurred speech
- Incoherence, indecisiveness
- Stupor or coma (this happens when body temperature goes below 90 F.)

Immediate Treatment

Mild Hypothermia
- Take temperature
- Prevent further cooling
- Warm up with any available means (sleeping bag, body to body, etc.)
- Keep victim moving and take to protected area
Severe Hypothermia
- Take temperature
- Prevent further cooling
- Keep very still
- Handle gently
- Rewarm slowly
- Find shelter
- Summon emergency help—if necessary, by helicopter

Prevention:

- Know the terrain
- Know predicted weather conditions
- Know the return trail
- Know your limits
- Know your companions
- Carry the following equipment (even for short climbs):

Extra socks, wool pants, wool sweaters, thermal underwear, parka, rain gear
Flashlight or headlight
First-aid kit
Extra food
Fire-starter material
Map of area
Compass
Sunglasses
Sunscreen
Thermometer

◆   Lightning

Every year an estimated one hundred people in the United States die from lightning strikes. Being aware of the danger will help you protect your youngster from this hazard during practice and competition, as well as at other times.

It's important for athletic directors, coaches, and trainers to become familiar with local weather patterns so they are better able to predict when lightning is possible. Specific responsibility should be assigned for deciding that a practice session or competitive event should be cancelled or halted. Procedures should be in place for the eventuality, such as:

1. If a lightning threat is present, the contest will be delayed for thirty minutes. If the threat has not diminished by that time, the game will be postponed and rescheduled.
2. Players and spectators will be directed to safe shelter.

Here are some basic guidelines to follow in case of lightning:

- Go indoors.
- Avoid open fields, but if in a field, lie down and curl up.
- Avoid single trees.
- If in an automobile, stay there.
- Avoid water, such as a pond, lake, river, etc.

PART III

Recognizing and Treating Sports Injuries

◆

8

Evaluating Sports Injury-Care Programs

◆

Being well-prepared to deal with sports injuries can ensure that all appropriate steps will be taken when an injury occurs. A detailed, well-documented plan of action must be in readiness—for youth-league programs, school programs, and individual-sports programs. Such a plan will minimize chances of further injury or complications caused by delay and confusion. The plan should provide not only for expediting care for the more common injuries but also for dealing with the rare severe accident—which means that the full capacity of the local medical community must be available.

◆ What Parents Should Know

Parents should get involved in sports-injury plans but generally don't. Here are some key questions you should ask about such plans:

- If an injury occurs, who will take care of it and where will the injured athlete be taken when more sophisticated care is needed?
- How well-qualified are those responsible for taking care of injuries?

- What are the plans for communication when an injury occurs?
- Is the necessary equipment on hand for injury care and emergencies?
- What are the procedures for returning the injured athlete to play after recovery?

There are also many other questions that parents should ask about the injury plan. Unfortunately, most parents don't get around to asking these questions until after an injury has occurred. In this chapter, we'll show how you can learn what you need to know *in advance*—and do something about any weak spots you find in an injury-care plan.

◆ SPORTS MEDICAL NIGHT FOR PARENTS

An orientation session for parents is a good way for you to learn about the injury-care plans of youth leagues or high-school athletic departments. If your youngster is participating in either type of sport and there is no such sports medical night, by all means suggest it to the appropriate officials. Such a program can also be organized by a local PTA (Parent-Teacher Association) group or a booster club made up of parents concerned about young people's sports.

Officials at the meeting should explain in detail plans made for any injury and the medical facilities that are available. In school sports, a tour of the training room and other sports-injury facilities can be informative. The session can also cover sports safety, physical examination requirements, and players' safety equipment. Coaches can explain their policies on attendance, scholastic requirements for eligibility, use of alcohol and drugs, discipline on the field, and other matters, as well as rules of the game and the safety responsibility of game officials. In a high-school program, all sports played should be covered.

This is an ideal opportunity for parents to ask any questions that concern them. Whether their attendance at the meeting is required or not, at least one parent from each family should be there.

The following guidelines for a sports medical night are geared toward school sports. However, the guidelines can be adapted for less elaborate meetings in youth-league sports.

Guidelines for a Sports Medical Night

A sports medical night should be held at the beginning of the season and should include all sports played during that season. At least one parent from each family and all coaches should be required to attend. The actual program should be planned and coordinated by the trainer and the team physician.

A comprehensive sports medical night should include these elements:

1. The meeting leader introduces all officials involved in each sport, with special attention to the trainers and their responsibilities.
2. Coaches hand out the rule books for each sport and review the rules specifically designed to minimize injuries.
3. Coaches explain their own disciplinary rules and regulations concerning such problems as use of alcohol and drugs.
4. Coaches describe their conditioning program and what conditioning exercises the young athletes are expected to do at home.
5. The trainer or coach recommends a home health program, including improved eating and sleeping habits.
6. The athletic director explains the specific plan of action followed when an injury occurs and also describes the medical care available in communities where "away" games are played.
7. Each family receives an information sheet with emergency telephone numbers, health insurance

and hospital information, and steps to be used in an emergency.

8. The trainer presents the contents of the trainer's bag and explains how each item is used.
9. The trainer or physician explains the risks of each sport, the typical injuries that occur, and specific care plans for a particular injury.
10. Coaches demonstrate the equipment worn for each sport and explain how it helps to prevent injuries. A good approach is to have a fully equipped player remove each piece of equipment as the coach explains its purpose.

◆ INJURY PLANS FOR YOUTH-LEAGUE SPORTS

Youth-league sports are generally quite safe, and serious injuries are uncommon among athletes under the age of thirteen. However, those in charge of these sports must be fully prepared to deal with the occasional serious injury or the rare catastrophe. At the start of a season, the directors should be ready with a formal plan for handling injuries and discuss it with all coaches and parents. In addition, the directors should distribute a printed copy of the plan at the meeting.

In most youth-league sports, coaches are responsible for taking care of an injury. A parent can withdraw an injured youngster from a game, but the coach has the final say on allowing an injured youngster to play. This approach normally works well.

Some teams will have parents who assume the role of team physician. Their specialty is unimportant—they may deliver babies—but they can take care of the bumps and bruises and refer parents to a specialist in the unusual case of a serious injury. If you know of a physician-parent on your youngster's team, ask if he/she would become a team "doc."

Any parent of a youth-league athlete should make sure

Checklist for an Effective Youth-League Injury Plan

Parents should ask the following questions about any sports program outside the school system, including programs in fitness and training centers.

1. *Is there a formal injury plan?*
2. *Is it in printed form?*
3. *Who has responsibility for injury care—coach or parent?*
4. *Does the coach have parents' home and work numbers?*
5. *Does the plan include emergency telephone numbers?*
6. *Are there provisions for emergency transportation?*
7. *Is there a well-stocked first-aid kit?*
8. *Who is responsible for water and ice?*
9. *Are the coaches qualified in CPR?*
10. *Have they taken a course in sports-injury prevention and care?*
11. *Do they have signed permission-for-care forms from parents so that when there is an emergency and no parent is present, a coach can obtain medical care for the injured youngster?*

that the playing facilities are safe. Courts, gyms, and fields run the gamut from sophisticated to primitive. Parents should expect the coach to take time before every game to survey the facilities for hazards that could cause injuries.

◆ INJURY PLANS FOR SCHOOL SPORTS

A well-coordinated school injury program involves a number of staff members with different responsibilities. You should have a clear picture of their roles and how they interact, so that in any injury situation involving your children you can contribute to the effectiveness of the program.

Here's what a typical sports medical team might look like:

Athletic Director

Coach   School Nurse

Trainer

Assistant Coach   Student Trainer

Team Physician

(School Physician)

Athletic Director

The athletic director is responsible for organizing the sports medical team so that it operates smoothly without panic in an emergency. Among the director's major injury-care duties are:

- To make sure all team members know their responsibilities, understand the plans for immediate action when an injury occurs, and are capable of carrying out specified procedures (which should be written and posted).
- To provide education for coaches in injury prevention and health maintenance.
- To keep injury records and information on all school sports safety policies.
- To ensure that there are adequate injury-care programs at other schools where away games are played. This includes checking to see that proper procedures are in place for handling injuries and that a physician and a hospital are available for medical emergencies.

Trainer

According to the American Academy of Orthopedic Surgeons, a trainer should have the following responsibilities:

1. Organizing and assuring proper medical care
2. Preventing and evaluating injuries
3. Making final decisions on whether a player can continue when an injury occurs and the team physician is not present
4. Providing care that does not require physician referral
5. Supervising, conditioning, and rehabilitating injured athletes
6. Educating staff and athletes on health care
7. Keeping records and maintaining protective equipment and medical supplies
8. Being able to perform cardiopulmonary resuscitation (CPR) when necessary

In fulfilling these duties, trainers rely on a team physician or sports medical specialist with whom they can communicate at any time. Trainers should always work under the guidance of this physician.

In practice, anyone can be *called* a trainer. However, trainers should only be considered qualified if they are either *certified* or *licensed*.

Trainers are certified by the National Athletic Trainers Association. Before qualifying for certification, they must have worked at least 1,500 hours with a certified trainer—and then must pass a written and practical examination. Some states license trainers using requirements that are usually similar to those used in NATA certification.

Any trainer hired by a school system should be qualified for CPR, emergency transportation, sports injury care, and post-injury evaluation and rehabilitation programming. No one should be allowed to function on the field or in the locker room as a trainer without meeting these qualifications. Too often, unqualified "trainers" miss the seriousness of a sports injury and make injury-care decisions beyond their expertise.

Ideally, of course, every school with interscholastic sports programs should have a professional athletic trainer. However, budgetary restrictions make this impossible for some schools. In that case, an assistant coach, a teacher, or a student trainer is an alternative, but only as a temporary expedient and when under the constant supervision of a physician. As soon as possible, the school should hire a professional trainer, preferably certified.

Coach

In many schools, the coach has prime responsibility for athletic injuries. This is not an ideal arrangement. Although most coaches do their best to make sound decisions on injuries, their appraisals may not be free from bias. Of course, most want strong, healthy players and excellent care of injuries. But they also want toughness, endurance, and fortitude. When it comes to deciding if an injured athlete should continue to play, they may make the wrong call. To ask them to make unbiased appraisals of injuries is neither fair to them nor to the injured student—these decisions should be made by a qualified trainer or team physician. However, even coaches with strong injury-care programs to back them up should be qualified to undertake emergency care, including CPR and basic first aid.

School Nurse

In schools without a professional trainer, the nurse may have overall responsibility for sports injuries, while the coach deals with them on the field. This is another less than ideal arrangement, because most school nurses have little expertise in sports medicine. Preferably, responsibility for injuries should be assigned to the athletic office, specifically to a certified trainer if there is one. The nurse's basic responsibility should be to monitor coordination between the athletic department and the school health office. Any nurse who does have responsibility for injuries should be required to take courses in sports medicine.

Team Physician

The team physician should have principal responsibility for coordinating the school's injury prevention efforts and care of injured athletes. The most effective team physicians get involved in the team's everyday activities and make themselves always available to the trainer, coach, athlete, and parents for advice. It is particularly comforting to parents to know that the physician is on the scene when their children are competing.

The team physician's top priority must be safety. Often that means being firm in the face of appeals to allow a young player to return to the field after being injured. In my twenty-five years as a high-school team physician, I have simply taken the helmet of any football player I felt should not return to the game. The coach immediately knew that youngster was out. Sometimes I might be holding three helmets, but both the coaches and the young athletes accepted this method of communication.

Some of a team physician's specific responsibilities are:

- Coordinating safety education programs with the trainer, such as staff education programs and a Parents' Sports Medical Night program
- Coordinating physical examinations for all school athletes
- Overseeing medical equipment and supplies in collaboration with the trainer
- Making sure medical care is available in other communities where away games are scheduled
- Attending all competitions that call for physician coverage (even when not required by law)

Most team physicians contribute their services out of an interest in young people and sports. They may be general physicians, orthopedic surgeons, or specialists in other disciplines. Often they stay with a school for many years, even though they may be paid nothing or only a small stipend.

Get to know the qualifications of your youngster's team physician. A team physician should be well educated in sports medicine and sports injuries, preferably through courses at the American College of Sports Medicine.

Make sure you know how to get in touch with the team physician when necessary. Be concerned about the team physician who shows up only for the game on Saturday but is never in the locker room or in contact with the trainer or coach between games.

◆ School Sports Medical Facilities

If you're the parent of a high-school athlete, take a sharp look at the school's medical facilities. Throughout the nation's high schools, these facilities can range from excellent to terrible. Some training rooms may be state-of-the-art while others are skimpy and antiquated. And yet top-class emergency equipment is essential if the school medical sports team is to function effectively.

Lack of money or unwillingness to spend it on sports medical facilities is often behind the poor facilities that exist. One problem is that parents generally don't get involved. They are seldom invited into the locker room or training room, so they don't even see the facilities for injury care. Parents should seek the opportunity to inspect the training room to make sure their young athletes are getting first-rate health care.

The Training Room

The training room is the center of all sports injury activity. Here is where injuries are checked and taped and post-injury treatment is initiated. This is the triage center where the trainer or physician makes decisions on the treatment of injuries. For example: Can the player return to action? Should the parents be called? Should the player be taken immediately to the hospital?

The training room houses student medical records and emergency telephone numbers for physicians and ambulances. All emergency first aid initiates from this room. It is also the communications center for team activities. Ideally, it should have a two-way radio system with communication between each playing field and the training room. As yet, this is a rarity.

What should a good training room be? It's important that it have a positive atmosphere. It should be well-located—not in a dingy corner of the school basement. It should be bright, clean, and organized, with sufficient space for both athletes and storage facilities. Emergency telephone numbers should be prominently posted (see pg 154). Trophies, posters, and team photographs will add to the winning edge.

Training Room Equipment

A good training room should include at least the following equipment:

General Facilities

- Clean room with good lighting
- Tables for examination and taping
- Hot and cold running water
- Scales
- Cabinets and/or shelves
- Physical therapy equipment such as a whirlpool

Emergency Equipment

- Trainer's field bag
- Oxygen and mask
- Stretcher
- Blankets
- Spine board or fracture board
- Crutches
- Fracture splints
- Sand bags to cushion injured areas

◆   Immediate Injury Care

A serious injury on the field can create havoc unless specific procedures have been set up for immediate, orderly

Emergency Telephone Numbers

These telephone numbers should be prominently posted in the training room:
- *Ambulance*
- *Police Department*
- *Fire Department*
- *Hospital*
- *Team Physician*
- *Specialists*
    - *Neurosurgeon*
    - *Ophthalmologist*
    - *Orthopedist*
    - *General Surgeon*
    - *Oral Surgeon*

Parent-notification numbers should be easily accessible in a well-organized file, including the following numbers:
- *First-call parent or guardian*
- *Second-call parent or guardian*
- *Other relative*

response. All personnel should be thoroughly indoctrinated in carrying out these procedures. Parents should make sure the following requirements are met by either a school athletic department or a youth-league team.

Clear Responsibility

During practice sessions and competition, each playing field should have a designated "field trainer" with immediate responsibility for injuries as soon as they occur. In most cases, this will be the coach or assistant coach. Whoever is assigned will carry out emergency action and direct immediate care until the trainer, ambulance, or physician arrives.

Well-Equipped Field Bag

That black bag you see on the sidelines at most inter-scholastic games is the emergency kit or trainer's field bag. It's the most important equipment for the immediate care of a sports injury—so it should contain every item that might be needed in an emergency.

Injury-Action Plan

A plan for *minor* injuries should include these steps:

* Determine that injury is minor (or player can be moved).
* Remove player to sidelines.
* Decide whether player can return to action or should go to locker room for treatment.
* Direct player to follow-up care, home, hospital, or specific physician.
* Record injury.
* Follow up on injury until resolved.

A plan for *major* injuries should include:

* Don't move athlete until injury has been evaluated.
* Determine athlete's basic condition:

A. Make sure airway is clear and breathing established.
B. Examine for bleeding and control it if necessary.
C. Check pulse to make sure circulation is present.

* Pinpoint injured part.
* Call for assistance, such as ambulance and/or physician.
* Protect injured part with splints, crutches, etc.
* Notify parents (and hospital, if necessary).

Intensity of pain at the moment of injury is usually the best immediate indicator of its severity. After the initial assessment and immediate first-aid measures, the next step can be determined. If the player can be moved, a qualified person should make a more complete assessment of the injury on the sidelines or in the training room (it is sometimes difficult to assess an injury on the field accurately). The responsible person can then decide whether to send the player home, to a hospital emergency room, or to a sports medical clinic.

If the player cannot be moved, an ambulance should be summoned. Back-up transportation—such as a station wagon—should always be available.

◆   The Perils of "Locker-Room" Medicine

"Locker-room" medicine can be dangerous and risky—sometimes serious injuries may be missed. Inexperienced trainers, student trainers, and others in the locker room may make decisions and give medical advice beyond their ability or training. They should be aware of their limitations and get the advice of a physician when an important medical decision must be made about an injured young athlete.

◆   INJURY PLANS FOR INDIVIDUAL SPORTS

Coaches for individual sports like gymnastics and skating should have their own injury-ready action program in writing. One source of confusion when injuries occur in individual sports is that managers of the facility the coach uses may have their own injury plan. That makes it important to coordinate plans and draw clear lines of responsibility for specific actions.

Like any coach, the individual-sports coach should have a well-stocked first-aid kit, a list of emergency numbers including parent-notification numbers, and certification for CPR. In addition, the coach should know what equipment is available in the facility for dealing with injuries.

Any facility that houses individual-sports activity—such as a gym, ice rink, or studio—should have its own well-organized plan for handling injuries. This should include:

1. Prominent posting of specific procedures to be followed in an emergency.
2. One person assigned to respond to an injury, who should be certified in CPR and preferably have taken an emergency medical training course.
3. The same person responsible for maintaining materials and supplies for emergencies—including a first-aid kit—which should be checked weekly.
4. List of emergency telephone numbers.
5. Information on the time required for an ambulance to respond to a call and transport an injured athlete to a hospital.

◆   INJURY PLANS IN SPORTS CAMPS

Sports camps for youngsters are becoming increasingly popular. Most of these camps are organized by coaches to train youngsters in specific sports. They can be sponsored by private operations, by religious organizations, or by high schools for their teams.

Summer day camps may be held at a local high school, prep school, or college. Their injury-care programs should meet the same standards discussed earlier.

Overnight camps present their own injury-care problems because your youngster may be far away from home for weeks. You should have two concerns: 1) your youngster's preparations for going away to sports camp, and 2) the quality of the camp's injury-care program.

◆   Preparations

Here's a checklist of questions that should help you prepare your youngster for sports camp:

1. Has your youngster passed a recent physical exam, and do you have a signed form to present to the camp?
2. Have there been any injuries or illnesses since the last examination? If so, a reexamination will be necessary.

3. Have you signed a permission slip for emergency care for your youngster?

4. Have you notified the camp about any special medications your youngster is taking?

5. Have you informed the camp about any health or activity restrictions on your youngster?

6. Does the camp know where you can be reached in an emergency?

7. Does your youngster have all the safety equipment required?

8. If there is a pre-camp training and conditioning program, has your youngster been following it?

9. Is your child enthusiastic about and emotionally prepared for the camp?

◆ Camp Injury-Care Plan

These are the questions you should ask about the camp's ability to cope with injuries:

1. Does the camp have an adequate program for dealing with emergencies?

2. Is it directed by a recognized leader or coach?

3. Are the facilities and buildings safe?

4. Is there a certified trainer always at the camp? If not, who is responsible for injuries?

5. Are camp personnel trained in CPR?

6. How many miles away is the nearest hospital?

7. Is the hospital prepared to handle injured youngsters from the camp?

8. Is there a physician available to deal with injuries at the camp?

To obtain further guidelines on injury-care plans for sports camps, write to the American Academy of Pediatrics, 151 Northwest Point Boulevard, Elk Grove Village, IL 60009.

◆ Sports Injuries at Camp

Most sports injuries at camp are not serious, with the exception of those at football camps. The most common problem is foot blisters caused by new sneakers—parents are embarrassed to send their youngster to camp with smelly old sneakers. Though not serious, these blisters can disable him or her for days, so be sure to send him or her to camp with sneakers that are already broken in. Two other problems are jock itch and athlete's foot, which can be prevented through cleanliness.

Injuries from hazing and initiation rites are more frequent in sports camps than in other types of camps. Be sure to express your concern to the camp director and find out what measures are taken to control such activities.

9

A Quick Home-Care Guide for 13 Everyday Sports Injuries

◆

Your young athlete *Jerry* comes home from a high-school wrestling match and you can see right away that he isn't feeling right. He reluctantly admits that he can't move his shoulder without a lot of pain—he must have injured it during the match. What should you do?

Often, care for a sports injury begins at home. In this case, Jerry never mentioned his injury to the team trainer—who might have done something about it if he had known. And this is a pattern for many youth injuries that occur in games and in practice: they are not reported to the trainer, coach, or doctor. The youngster may not think the injury amounts to much or may keep quiet about it for fear of being benched.

So it's up to you to provide the immediate care of the injury and to seek professional medical care if it is needed. This guide will help you deal with thirteen common types of injuries that your youngsters are likely to bring home.

◆   **GENERAL HOME CARE**

First, how will you know an injury has occurred? Your youngster won't necessarily tell you—it's one of the endearing traits of kids to clam up about these things. Consider *Kathy*. She comes home from basketball practice and says nothing about any injury. But she's quiet and withdrawn—and defensively denies that anything's wrong. That's your cue that she may have injured herself at practice and is in possibly severe pain. If she's unwilling to tell you what's wrong, you should insist on taking her to a physician.

Many of the injuries your youngsters bring home will not require immediate medical attention. If an injury seems to be minor according to the guidelines in this chapter, just observe it overnight to make sure there is nothing seriously wrong. Whisking your youngster to the emergency room for every little bump and bruise simply overloads already crowded medical facilities for no good reason. You can usually take care of the simple first-aid measures yourself.

◆ Exceptions to Waiting

When your gut feeling tells you the injury is more severe or you are simply worried about it, it's best to check with a doctor.

Some clues that indicate you should seek immediate help are:

- Severe pain.
- Massive swelling.
- Severe tenderness to the touch.
- Inability to use an arm.
- An injury to the head or eye—NEVER take chances with such injuries.

◆ Applying the RICE Procedure

There are certain basic first-aid measures you should take with your youngster no matter where the injury is located.

Injuries seen at home on the same day they occurred should receive some or all of four types of treatment known throughout the sports world as the RICE procedure: rest, ice, compression, and elevation (not necessarily in that order).

1. *Rest.* Get your youngster into a comfortable position, either sitting or lying down. If there is severe pain, put the injured part in a sling or cardboard splint (wrap an injured leg or ankle in a pillow). Then try to get your youngster to rest. This may not be easy, of course, but rest is still the first and best healer.
2. *Ice.* Place soft, crushed ice in a plastic bag and apply it directly to the painful, swollen area. Try to mold it around the part that hurts. Commercial ice packs may be used as well. But whatever you use, always be sure it's something cold—never apply heat to a fresh injury.
3. *Compression.* Swelling can be limited by applying an elastic bandage to the injured part (if you have active youngsters, it's a good idea to always have these bandages on hand).
4. *Elevation.* Put the injured part higher than the heart, so it will not swell as much. The less swelling, the faster the healing.

Here's an example of the RICE procedure. Compression: Wrap a sprained ankle with an elastic bandage from the toes to well above the ankle, using comfortable pressure. Elevation and rest: Elevate the ankle on a pillow with the youngster lying down so that the ankle is higher than the heart. Ice: Pack a large amount of soft ice in a plastic bag around the ankle and keep it that way for several hours or overnight. This procedure will usually minimize the damage from your youngster's injury.

◆   **Your Home First-Aid Kit**

To provide simple care for the normal cuts, bruises, and aches and pains of your youngsters' sports activities, keep the following items in your home first-aid kit:

1. Adhesive bandages: six or more, 1″ size
2. Gauze pads: six 3″, six 4″

3. Gauze bandage: one or two 2″ rolls
4. Adhesive tape: a 1″ roll and a 2″ roll
5. Antiseptic solution (Betadine)
6. Elastic bandages: two 3″, two 4″
7. Cream for sunburn
8. Triangular bandage for a sling
9. Over-the-counter pain medicine, such as aspirin

◆ QUICK HOME-CARE GUIDES FOR 13 COMMON SPORTS INJURIES

How to Use This Section: The guides that follow are for thirteen common types of sports injuries that your youngster may bring home, classified by parts of the body: *head, neck, shoulder, elbow, wrist, hand, back, hip, thigh, knee, leg, ankle, and foot.* When your youngster comes home with any of these injuries, flip to the guide covering it and follow the recommended measures for immediate care.

These guides are limited to immediate home care of everyday complaints of youngsters who engage in competitive sports. Chapters 13–17 discuss a broad range of more specific injuries in greater detail. Following each of the thirteen immediate-care guides in this chapter you will find page numbers for the more detailed information on the particular type of injury being discussed.

Each quick-care guide suggests next steps to take after immediate treatment has been given. In some cases, these will include getting medical help, either immediately or within a day or two. If you think your young athlete needs to see a physician, stick to your guns even if your youngster objects. This is a common-sense call.

1. Head Injuries

COMPLAINT
"I had my bell rung."
"I had a ding."
"I had a concussion."

SYMPTOMS

Mild headache. If there has been any loss of consciousness, change in vision, or nausea, the youngster should go right to the hospital.

HOME CARE

Rest at home, aspirin or over-the-counter pain pill. The youngster should not go out.

NEXT STEPS

No matter how mild it seems, *every head injury must be taken seriously.* Of all injuries, head injuries are the least likely to show obvious signs of trouble. Therefore, even when the symptoms are mild, a next-day diagnosis by a physician is imperative.
For more detailed information on head injuries, see pages 196–198.

2. Neck Injuries

COMPLAINT

"I have a stiff neck."
"I had a burner."
"I had a stinger."

SYMPTOMS

Stiff neck with pain, and possibly numbness or arm tingling.

HOME CARE

Rest lying down, head on a pillow. Apply ice or a cold, wet washcloth. Also administer aspirin or an over-the-counter pain pill.

NEXT STEPS

Not usually a serious injury in young athletes. However, if there is severe pain or arm tingling and numbness, the injury should be checked by a doctor the next day.

For more detailed information on neck injuries, see pages 199–204.

3. Shoulder Injuries

COMPLAINT

"I can't raise my arm."
"My shoulder popped."
"My shoulder hurts."

SYMPTOMS

A sore, possibly swollen shoulder that hurts to move.

HOME CARE

Apply ice, put the arm in a sling, and make your youngster take it easy. He or she will be more comfortable sitting and letting the shoulder hang loosely. If you're not using a sling, the arm should be bent by resting it on a chair arm.

NEXT STEPS

Most shoulder injuries can be checked medically the following day. However, if there is severe pain, take your youngster to an emergency room that day.
For more detailed information on shoulder injuries, see pages 211–223.

4. Elbow Injuries

COMPLAINT

"My elbow hurts."

SYMPTOMS

Swelling about the elbow, but the elbow motion is good.

HOME CARE

Apply ice and make the youngster rest.

NEXT STEPS

Most elbow injuries are not serious and do not call for immediate medical attention. But if there is severe pain and swelling, or the elbow can't be moved without severe pain, consult a physician without delay, because there could be a fracture.

For more detailed information on elbow injuries, see pages 223–233.

5. Wrist Injuries

COMPLAINT

"I sprained my wrist."

SYMPTOMS

Pain, possible swelling.

HOME CARE

Rest, ice, elastic bandage, and elevation.

NEXT STEPS

As mentioned earlier, every wrist injury should be considered a fracture until proven otherwise. The problem could be a fracture of the *navicular* bone, the most frequently overlooked serious fracture in an athlete. So when your youngster comes home saying, "I sprained my wrist," *don't accept that description until a fracture has been ruled out.* Although emergency action is not necessary, the wrist must be X-rayed within the next two days. Even if no fracture is seen, repeat in ten to fourteen days to confirm the original finding.

For more detailed information on wrist injuries, see pages 233–236.

6. Hand Injuries

COMPLAINT

"I jammed my finger."
"I sprained my finger."
"My hand hurts."

SYMPTOMS

Swelling of the knuckles, fingers, or whole hand.

HOME CARE

Apply ice, elevate the hand, and put on a finger splint, if available.

NEXT STEPS

Not an emergency, but the injury must be seen by a physician to make sure it is not a fracture or ligament rupture.

For more detailed information on hand injuries, see pages 237–245.

7. Back Injuries

COMPLAINT

"My back hurts."

SYMPTOMS

Low back pain, stiffness. It hurts to sit and bend over, and the youngster can't tie shoes or get out of a chair.

HOME CARE

Rest lying down, ice, and aspirin or over-the-counter pain medicine.

NEXT STEPS

Probably not serious, but if there is any leg pain or numbness, seek medical attention the next day.

For more detailed information on back injuries, see pages 253–260.

8. Hip Injuries

COMPLAINT

"I have a hip pointer."
"I have a groin pull."
"I sprained my hip."

SYMPTOMS

Stiffness, limping, and soreness in the groin or side of hip.

HOME CARE

Rest, ice. Okay to limp around unless the pain is too severe.

NEXT STEPS

Have your youngster seen by a doctor if he or she limps for more than a few days—there may be a serious condition. X rays are essential for diagnosis.

For more detailed information about hip injuries, see pages 264–270.

9. Thigh Injuries

COMPLAINT

"I have a charley horse."
"I pulled a hamstring."

SYMPTOMS

Thigh pain, swelling, and a stiff knee joint. Back of the thigh is painful.

HOME CARE

Rest, ice, and compression. Do *not* use heat.

NEXT STEPS

If the pain is severe and the thigh is very swollen, get immediate medical attention.

For more information about thigh injuries, see pages 270–275.

10. Knee Injuries

COMPLAINT

"I twisted my knee."
"I sprained my knee."
"My knee feels weird."

SYMPTOMS

Limping and swelling, and the knee may give way.

HOME CARE

Rest, ice. Apply an elastic bandage from three inches below to three inches above the kneecap and place the leg on a pillow.

NEXT STEPS

Knee injuries can be serious and disabling. Have an orthopedic surgeon examine the knee as soon as possible, because once the swelling and pain become severe, an examination may require anesthesia.

For more information about knee injuries, see pages 298–329.

11. Leg Injuries

COMPLAINT

"I have a shin splint."

SYMPTOMS

Pain in the front or side. It hurts to walk. Swelling is rare and there is usually no visible injury.

HOME CARE

Rest, ice.

NEXT STEPS

Leg pains are usually a nuisance condition. But when there is severe pain in the front of the leg, immediate medical care is necessary to prevent permanent damage. Don't guess—go.

For more information about leg injuries, see pages 275–281.

12. Ankle Injuries

COMPLAINT

"I sprained my ankle."
"My ankle popped."

SYMPTOMS

Swelling around the outside of the ankle bone. The ankle may turn black-and-blue within twelve to twenty-four hours. Pain, with severity depending on amount of ligament damage.

HOME CARE

Rest, ice, compression with elastic bandage, and elevation.

NEXT STEPS

An ankle sprain is not an emergency. However, good care for the first major ankle injury is critical. If proper healing does not take place, the ankle may remain loose and unstable. An orthopedic surgeon should determine the treatment of ankle injuries.
For more information about ankle injuries, see pages 281–285.

13. Foot Injuries

COMPLAINT

"I sprained my foot."

SYMPTOMS

Limping, some swelling, possible tenderness at a specific point.

HOME CARE

Rest, ice, compression with an elastic bandage.

NEXT STEPS

If your youngster has severe pain and can't walk on the injured foot, get immediate medical attention. Otherwise, wait until the next day—if there's no improvement by then, see a physician to make sure there's no fracture.

For more information about foot injuries, see pages 285–297.

10

Getting Good Medical Care

◆

Minor sports injuries usually need no more care than first aid on the field and later treatment at home, as described in the previous chapter. But more serious injuries may require emergency-room care and the services of a sports medical specialist, possibly including surgery. Let's hope it won't happen to your child. But if it does, you should be prepared by knowing how to get good medical care for your injured athlete.

◆ **THE EMERGENCY ROOM**

Any time an injured young athlete must be taken to an emergency room, an adult—preferably the coach, trainer, or parent—should go along to provide psychological support and tell the emergency room doctor what happened.

Emergency-room care should be just that—taking care of the immediate emergency and leaving long-term decisions to a pediatrician, orthopedic surgeon, or sports medical specialist. The emergency room should definitely *not* be where final decisions on the seriousness of sports injuries are made.

172

◆ THE SPORTS MEDICAL SPECIALIST

Sports injuries and sports-related medical problems are best cared for by a sports medical specialist if one is available. Most sports physicians are orthopedic surgeons—and because most injuries to young athletes are orthopedic in nature, I believe that an orthopedic surgeon should be involved in the primary diagnosis and early-care planning of a youth sports injury. Initial care is critical. Sports physicians may also be pediatricians, neurosurgeons, osteopaths, ophthalmologists, pulmonary (lung) physicians, psychologists, or psychiatrists. Nonphysicians specializing in sports can be nutritionists, certified trainers, podiatrists, or exercise physiologists.

Although there are many more sports medical specialists today than there were ten years ago, you still won't find one on every corner, so you may have to travel some distance for a consultation. Another difficulty is that some HMOs, comprehensive care centers, and medical insurance companies do not allow a patient to go directly to a sports medical specialist rather than to a primary-care physician. This is in the interest of cutting costs, but a primary-care physician who undertakes to treat sports injuries instead of referring youngsters to a sports medical specialist may not be expert enough always to diagnose and treat them correctly. An incorrect diagnosis can delay proper care, with serious results. I have seen some disturbing cases: a severe leg injury that went unrecognized, resulting in permanent paralysis; a dislocated knee that was undiscovered for two weeks; and a major ligament injury to the knee that was completely missed.

◆ Selecting a Sports Medical Specialist

If you need the advice of a specialist in athletic injuries, use care in selecting one. Don't assume that all health-care practitioners who list themselves as sports medical specialists are really qualified—many of them are not. However, there are some guidelines that can help you select one who is. Try to find one who:

- Participates in a local sports medical education program
- Has attended sports medical courses
- Is a team physician for a local school team or is active in youth-league programs
- Devotes a substantial amount of time to caring for athletes
- If an orthopedic surgeon, is a fellow of the American Orthopedic Society for Sports Medicine
- Is a member of the American College of Sports Medicine
- Was an athlete as a youth and is still active in sports

What if there is no sports medical specialist available to you? In that case, you might consult your family physician or local hospital for advice on where to go for good care. There are usually orthopedic surgeons and physicians in every area who can handle most sports injuries even though they are not sports specialists.

◆   What the Specialist Should Explain

You should leave the office of a sports medical specialist—or any physician—with a good understanding of your youngster's injury, a clear picture of what to expect from the injury, and all of the options available for treatment. Make sure you get this information from the physician and not from the physician's assistant or other aide.

Although simple, routine injuries don't require exhaustive diagnosis and discussion, others must be explained and diagrammed in great detail to give you and your youngster the complete facts. A good specialist will allow you time to absorb the situation so you can make an educated decision on further action.

◆   Difficulties With Parents

As a sports medical specialist and father of eight children who have had their share of sports injuries, I can sympathize with the anxious parents who bring their youngsters to my office. Nevertheless, I ask to see the youngster alone. Why? Because I know that I can find out more about the youngster's complaints without the presence of parents. With parents listening, most teenagers clam up. Or they look to the parents for answers to my questions. Then there are parents who don't even give the youngster a chance to talk—they jump in with answers to my questions for the injured athlete. For example, if I ask a youngster "Where does it hurt?" a parent immediately says, "It hurts him right here, doctor, in the elbow."

Some parents won't accept the fact that their presence is a hindrance rather than a help. I've heard the familiar responses many times:

"I want to be in the room to make sure he tells you everything."

"I don't trust him."

"She won't say anything if I'm not there."

"I want to know what's going on."

If a parent insists on being in the room when I examine a youngster, I don't object. However, I strongly recommend that parents refrain from insisting unless they have solid reasons. It is important that youngsters learn to take responsibility for their own bodies and the injuries that may occur.

◆ When It's a Question of Surgery

A serious injury to your youngster may require surgery. If you have any doubts about your doctor's recommendations either for or against surgery, don't be afraid to get a second opinion from another reputable athletic surgeon. No professionally secure physician will object to your consulting another doctor or even to your deciding to follow the second doctor's recommendation.

Your doctor should clearly explain the options and risks involved—both immediate and long-term. In most cases, there will be no disagreement. For example, most sports medical specialists agree that surgery is the best way to

Dealing With Injured Youngsters—A Holistic Approach

In treating youngsters with sports injuries I try to deal with the whole person, not just the physical injury. My first interview with the young patient includes questions about brothers, sisters, grades, parents, the school year, activities, interests outside of sports, how much they really enjoy the sport they're in, what position they play, and so on. I get a fix on their anxieties, their attitude toward coaches, their feelings about winning and losing, and peer pressure. This is one reason I prefer to see these youngsters without their parents in the room during the first interview. For example, one boy's father told me that his son was interested only in baseball—but when I talked to the youngster alone he told me, "I'd rather play golf than baseball."

Only when I have built a good foundation do I start discussing the youngster's specific injury in terms of seriousness, choices of treatment, timing of return to play, and so on. I make it clear to youngsters that this is not just something for other people to decide, that they must take responsibility for dealing with the injury—and if it does not feel right to them, they should not play, regardless of what I say. That's not easy when you're dealing with a teenager, but it's much easier if a rapport has been established.

correct a chronic dislocating shoulder. With some injuries, however, sports surgeons may legitimately disagree as to the need for surgery. There are two distinct schools of thought on separated shoulders, for example. One favors operating to reduce the separation, using a screw or wire. The other maintains that separated shoulders can be healed nonsurgically with a harness that closes the separation.

Knee surgery presents another difficult decision. Again, if you have any doubts about your first doctor's recommendation, don't hesitate to get another opinion so you can carefully consider the options and risks.

When two doctors disagree on the wisest course for your youngster, you'll be faced by a troublesome situation to which there is no easy answer. All you can do is educate yourself—and your youngster—on all the pros and cons of each recommended procedure. Choose the surgeon who seems to make the best sense. Don't hesitate to ask questions and get specific reasons for the surgeon's recommendations.

◆ DEALING WITH X RAYS

Are X rays necessary for diagnosing sports injuries? Absolutely. More than thirty years of practicing sports medicine have convinced me that without X rays many serious injuries will go unrecognized, with sometimes disastrous consequences.

Although X rays are not foolproof, the actual extent of an injury can rarely be determined without one. For, example, an X ray may show that:

- A seemingly mild head injury is a depressed fracture of the skull.
- A shoulder injury is hiding a fracture.
- A "wrist sprain" is actually a dangerous navicular fracture.
- A knee sprain is a growth-line fracture.
- A seemingly simple shin splint is a stress fracture.

◆ But Aren't X Rays Dangerous?

Research studies show that some risk must be assumed even with small amounts of radiation. However, most experts agree that the benefits of *necessary* X rays outweigh the risks. Every parent should be constantly vigilant against unnecessary radiation exposure, even in its lowest form.

◆ Minimizing X-Ray Exposure

What can you do to minimize X-ray exposure while maximizing medical care for your injured youngster? Asking the following questions of your doctor will help:

1. *Why is this X ray necessary and what will it tell?* Ask your doctor to give you a full explanation of his or her reasons for taking an X ray.
2. *What method of radiation protection will be used?* For genitals and female breasts, clinics should use a full body apron or lead sheets covering at least the breasts and pelvis.
3. *How many exposures will be taken?* Exposures should be kept to the absolute minimum necessary. For example, although many doctors take three views in a routine study, two may be enough.
4. *Does the X-ray machine have an inspection certificate?* No X-ray machine should be used unless it has passed a required safety inspection by the state. The inspection certificate must be posted in the X-ray area.
5. *How old is the X-ray machine?* New machines have screening devices to reduce the amount of exposure to the minimum necessary. Find out if the machine that will be used for your youngster has this device.
6. *Are the walls of the X-ray room properly shielded?* The walls should have $\frac{1}{16}$-inch-thick lead shielding to protect other areas of the clinic from radiation.

◆ Keeping an X-Ray Exposure Record

Keep an accurate record of all X rays taken of your youngster. Then you will know exactly how many X rays your young athlete has had rather than constantly worrying whether he or she has had too many. A convenient way to keep these records is provided by the *Child Health Record* booklet available from the American Academy of Pediatrics, 151 Northwest Point Boulevard, Elk Grove Village, IL 60009.

Other Diagnostic Aids

Other tools besides X rays can be useful in diagnosing orthopedic sports injuries. When X rays do not provide for a satisfactory diagnosis, your doctor may recommend one of the following tests: bone scan, image intensifier (MRI), CAT scan, liver and spleen scan, or ultrasound.

◆   Should Parents Look At X Rays?

I say, "Why not?" But only in the presence of the doctor, who can explain what you're looking at. Don't try to read X rays on your own. You'll be alarmed by seeing things that are actually quite normal ("Good God, what's that big black thing?") and pleased to see an apparently healed fracture that really hasn't healed. I have to laugh when a father looks over my shoulder at an X ray and says, "It looks okay to me, Doc!" What he's really saying is, "He can play, can't he?" It takes many years of experience to interpret these X rays and determine how much healing has taken place. Rely on the physician to decide if your youngster is ready to play in the next game or even that season.

11

Guiding Your Youngster Through the "Injury Interaction"

◆

Dick is an 18-year-old quarterback for his high-school football team, which is hoping to win the state championship this year. When he pops his knee in practice, the team physician tells him he's out for the season. How are his teammates and other students going to take this?

Melanie is a track star about to compete at the Dartmouth Relays for national recognition. Two days before the meet, she sprains her foot while training. How will she respond emotionally to being unable to compete?

Pete is a third-string hockey player on his high-school team. While checking another player during practice, he suffers a separated shoulder. Will his teammates care?

Hundreds of such injuries occur every day throughout the United States. Many of them involve not just a physical injury, but an emotional one as well. The youngster's recovery from the psychological trauma depends largely on the responses of those most closely involved: parents, coach, trainer, physician, and friends. I call these contacts with the young athlete *injury interactions*.

A sports injury to a youngster can generate a tangle of emotional reactions, sometimes obvious, but often hidden. They may be easy to manage or create serious problems that are difficult to resolve. Do your best to understand how the injury is affecting your youngster so that you can be as supportive and helpful as possible.

Usually involved are the youngster's feelings of personal value and self-confidence, as well as relations with people in his or her immediate world. The athlete's response to the injury depends greatly on the circumstances and background, which can vary widely. For example:

- The injury may be indirectly related to internal turmoil over family problems or other adolescent anxieties.
- The injury may occur during practice with no one else aware of its severity.
- It may occur in a big game when everyone was depending on the athlete's performance.
- Or it may occur early in the season before a young athlete has ever had a chance to shine.
- The injury may be related to a careless mistake or a rules violation, in which case it could have been avoided. (In many instances, only the young athlete knows what happened.)
- In individual sports, the injury might result from an error— such as a hand slip on the uneven bars in gymnastics—after years of training.

Whatever the circumstances, an understanding of injury interactions can help you in trying to ease your injured youngster's emotional stress. Others involved—such as the coach, the trainer, the youngster's peers, and the treating physician—can also help. However, you can't depend on this, so you must be ready to provide the support and comfort that your youngster needs.

◆ THE COACH

Coaches have several priorities, including winning, so they may react in many different ways to an injured athlete: acceptance, support, understanding, indifference, frustration, anxiety, anger, threat, fear are some of the possible responses. In the heat of battle or preparation for a big game, a coach under stress may respond unsympathetically when a valuable player is injured. If the injury is to a third-string player, the coach may simply ignore the young athlete.

Whatever the coach's response, it will register strongly on the injured youngster, and can help or hinder recovery. At this crucial time, the coach should provide support and reassurance, whether the young athlete is a star player or a seldom-used substitute.

One thing that can help when a youngster has been injured is a good interaction between parent and coach. Unfortunately, animosity may develop. Some parents may blame the coach for the injury. Others may feel the coach didn't pay enough attention to the injury when it occurred. Some parents with a different mind-set may blame the coach for benching their youngster when they think he or she is able to play. In response, the coach may be resentful of parental "interference."

Two-way understanding is key here. By establishing a good rapport with the coach and recognizing the coach's concerns and responsibilities, parents can ease a situation that could easily worsen the emotional impact of the injury. The coach can be sensitive to the parents' anxieties and misgivings and try to relieve them as much as possible.

◆ THE TRAINER

If the trainer has your youngster's confidence, this interaction can be pivotal in helping the youngster to develop a healthy perspective on the injury. In the first few moments after the injury occurs, a trainer's understanding can make a big difference. The young athlete's ego has been hurt along with his or her body, so support and reassurance are badly needed at this point and later. The trainer can ease disappointment and anxiety by discussing the treatment and explaining why it takes a certain length of time to heal. A good trainer's care can help to speed recovery and strengthen the injured youngster's confidence.

◆ PEERS

Supportive reactions from teammates and friends can help the injured youngster emotionally. But negative reactions can be terribly hurtful. If the youngster is an outstanding competitor, there may be remarks like:

"Well, there goes the season."

"She's the only one who can score."

"Nobody can throw like him."

If the injured player isn't that valuable, the attitude is often indifference. Either way, the young athlete feels rejected, not a happy condition for anyone, much less a sensitive teenager. If you're aware of this situation, a frank conversation about it with your youngster can lighten the burden and relieve some internal pressure.

◆ YOU AS PARENTS

Probably the most important interaction of all is between your injured youngster and you. Your attitude can make a key difference in the way your young athlete copes with the injury. This is particularly true if it's a serious injury that will take weeks or months to heal.

So be sure that what you say does not make the situation worse rather than better. Above all, avoid blame. Some parents react with accusations:

"You just blew a four-year scholarship!"

"You're the best pitcher they've got—what happened to you, dummy, you never get hurt!"

"The other boy hit you on purpose!"

Try to be reassuring and positive—but also be realistic. Don't raise false hopes by saying, "It's nothing—you'll be back playing tomorrow," when the recovery will take much longer than that. There are times when you have to say very little—just a simple hug or pat on the back will raise your youngster's spirits. At other times you may see the need for a good long talk at the kitchen table. *To sum up*: Listen to your youngster and be generous with your support, reassurance, and understanding.

◆ THE PHYSICIAN

When parents take their injured youngster to a physician, the prevailing mood is understandably anxiety. You may be worried about permanent effects of the injury, while your youngster may be concerned about returning to competition as soon as possible. The interaction here can be a major step in recovery from the injury. The physician should be sensitive to the psychological elements of the injury as well as the purely physical problem, and try to deal with both. By recognizing the entire injury interaction, the physician can give the parents and their youngster the strength to accept the fact of the injury and what must be done to recover from it, even when it means not being able to compete for a while.

◆ THE FINAL INTERACTION

This interaction usually takes place when it's time to decide if an injured youngster is ready to return to competition or perhaps should be eliminated from competing altogether because of the injury. These decisions must come in writing from the responsible physician, whether the team physician, school doctor, family doctor, or sports medical specialist. The coach or trainer should not assume responsibility for making an important decision for which he or she is not medically qualified. And parents, in their turn, should be prepared to accept the doctor's decision as well. The worst scenario is when a parent says, "I don't care what the doctor says—he's my child and I'm going to permit him to play." That's risking disaster for the young athlete.

The way in which the return-to-competition decision is handled can be helpful or hurtful to the youngster's emotional well-being. If a decision against return is handed down as a brusque ultimatum, the youngster's morale may sink to zero. It's important for all the adults involved in the decision to discuss it openly with the youngster, clearly explain why return to competition is inadvisable, and suggest alternatives.

12

Long-Term Consequences of Sports Injuries

◆

There's a crying need for solid information on the long-term effects of sports injuries incurred by young athletes, yet very little has been written on the subject. Many parents are understandably concerned about the problem. They themselves may have suffered injuries in their youth that left permanent consequences, and they don't want it to happen to their kids. At the same time, there are also many parents who believe the value of sports far outweighs the dangers. Whatever your own attitude, you should know about the difficulties that may be encountered in later years from certain sports injuries.

Children rarely suffer any permanent sports injuries before the age of fourteen. In fact, while treating young athletes for more than thirty years, I have encountered only a small number of cases. Two were knee injuries, one from motorcycle racing, the other from downhill skiing. And despite the talk about permanent injuries to the growth centers of young bones, I have seen only two: a wrist fracture and an ankle fracture. Neither injury limited the youngster in later life. Of course, the trend toward more strenuous competition among younger players may increase the number of injuries with lasting effects. But even in collision sports such as football, soccer, hockey, and wrestling, the elasticity of the young body makes serious injuries relatively rare. And when opposing teams are well-balanced, there is not enough force in the collision of two young bodies to cause much damage. Recreational bike riding is far more dangerous than competitive sports to youngsters under fourteen.

The real threat of permanent injuries starts at the high-school level. The following guide discusses the more common long-term injuries, their significance, and the sports in which they are most likely to occur. These injuries are described more fully in the *Home Reference Guide*.

◆ WHAT INJURIES CAUSE PERMANENT DISABILITIES?

FACE

Injuries leaving scars mostly occur to the face from sticks and pucks, as well as direct head blows in such sports as soccer, basketball, and diving. Even with full helmets, football has its share of permanent scars from lacerations. They also occur in skiing from falling or hitting obstacles. The loss of front teeth has been reduced by mouth guards and face masks, but sometimes occurs even when they are worn. Cauliflower ears are a permanent cosmetic injury seen in wrestling.

Most unattractive scars can be minimized through expert reconstructive surgery.

HEAD

In youth sports, most head injuries do not cause permanent damage. On average, three permanent head injuries occur annually in high-school football in the United States. The incidence in other sports is probably even lower. In boxing, head injuries can leave long-term consequences, but there is no evidence that a young amateur boxer who stops the sport after the age of nineteen will suffer any residual damage.

EYES

Decreased vision or loss of sight can occur from injuries in hockey, racquet sports, and lacrosse.

NECK

One of the greatest tragedies in sports is the neck injury that causes permanent paralysis. This takes two forms: *quadriplegia*, complete paralysis from the neck down; and *paraplegia*, paralysis of the legs. This injury is most commonly caused by diving into shallow water—over seven hundred youngsters are paralyzed each year from diving accidents. Spearing in football also causes a significant number of paralyzing injuries, but far fewer than diving. Such injuries can also occur in hockey and gymnastics. The only answer to these injuries is prevention.

On a less serious level, repeated neck injuries in collision or impact sports can result in long-term cervical arthritis, causing occasional periods of a painful, stiff neck and sometimes a pinched nerve with pain running into the arm or shoulder. These periods recur most often in one's fifties and sixties, but can start earlier. This long-term problem occurs frequently in football, wrestling, hockey, and rugby.

BACK

Back injuries from sports are rarely permanent. The exception is a condition called *spondylolisthesis* in young gymnasts and football players. This can be a life-time problem that restricts recreational sports after one's late twenties or early thirties. It may require orthopedic care over the years, and sometimes surgery.

CHEST

Injuries along the rib cage and chest-plate may leave a permanent bump, but no discomfort or disability.

SHOULDER

A serious shoulder injury incurred in teenage sports is one of the injuries most likely to come back and haunt the athlete in later life. Separations may frequently cause pain and discomfort later, while rotator-cuff injuries, though uncommon before the age of nineteen, can cause the most long-term trouble. These problems can make throwing painful as early as the thirties. Moreover, they are often aggravated in middle age by activities such as tennis, carpentry, and gardening. In some cases, surgery is required to relieve the pain.

Shoulder injuries with life-long disability are most likely to occur in high-school baseball, softball, football, swimming, wrestling, gymnastics, lacrosse, and hockey.

ELBOW

Although elbow problems are common in youth-league baseball, they seldom cause difficulties in later life. The only exceptions are *osteochondritic* damage and avulsion fractures from throwing, and these long-term problems are uncommon.

WRIST

Most wrist injuries leave no permanent effects. However, if a *navicular* fracture is overlooked and not treated promptly, the wrist joint can develop painful, disabling arthritis. This injury occurs most commonly in roller-skating, football, and hockey, but can happen with a fall in any sport.

HANDS AND FINGERS

Although these injuries can leave thick joints and stiffness in the fingers, most people adjust quite easily. However, ligament injuries to the thumb may leave a weak grip if not repaired surgically, and mallet fingers may result in a loose fingertip.

KNEE

Of all sports injuries to young people, knee injuries are most likely to cause permanent damage and disabling pain. Although there have been remarkable advances in knee surgery, this is still *the* number one long-term sports injury problem. The worst consequences stem from damage to the *anterior cruciate ligament.* Other common problems with possible long-term effects are dislocated kneecaps, torn *meniscus* (cartilage), and *osteochondritis*. Degenerative arthritis may develop from these injuries, although it is impossible to predict the extent—it depends on the severity of the injury, the abuse received by the knee afterwards, and whether a ligament reconstruction, if done, will help to reduce the arthritis.

Knee injuries can occur in any sport, but most often in skiing, field hockey, football, basketball, soccer, moto-cross, wrestling, hockey, and lacrosse.

ANKLE

Few ankle injuries cause permanent disability, although ankle fractures can lead to arthritis. After repeated ankle injuries, spurs may form, but they respond well to surgical excision. Looseness of the ankle can be mildly disabling.

Ankle injuries occur in every sport, but most often in basketball, volleyball, baseball, soccer, gymnastics, football, tennis, squash, and track and field.

FOOT

Foot injuries with permanent effects are rare. The most common is arthritis from "turf toe," which can be relieved by surgery. Fractures that don't heal can also be corrected surgically, leaving little residual disability. Several congenital foot conditions can be aggravated by overuse, and in later years may require medical care. Foot injuries are frequently reported in martial arts, skating, swimming, and track and field.

PART IV

Home Reference Guide to Sports Injuries—From Head to Toe

◆

About This Guide

◆

In this guide you will find practical information about specific injuries that your young athlete might suffer. These injuries range from commonplace to rare, and from superficial to severe. Fractures that are routine orthopedic problems not specific to sports are not discussed. Stress fractures, however, are fully covered.

Consult this guide whenever your youngster has an injury from sports. If the youngster comes home with the injury, refer first to Chapter 9: *A Quick Home-Care Guide for 13 Everyday Sports Injuries*. Then go to the *Home Reference Guide* for more information about the injury.

The information in the *Home Reference Guide* will help you to understand the injury and its cause, recognize the symptoms, know when to take your youngster to a physician, discover ways to prevent it, and learn about the preferred treatment.

For each injury you will find recommendations on when the young athlete can return to competition. There are no absolute rules for determining this—it depends on many variables, including the ability of the individual athlete to respond to an injury, the particular sport, the athlete's status on the team, and the athlete's mental attitude.

It's my belief that a physician should evaluate all these factors before deciding on return to play. When viewed in perspective, an injury may not necessarily prevent a young athlete from competing.

This doesn't mean that the physical injury itself mustn't be carefully evaluated. A physician should only say "OK to go" when the young athlete has recovered sufficiently to return to competition without serious danger of further problems from this particular injury.

However, equally important is the attitude of the injured athlete. The confident athlete is less likely to be reinjured than one who is insecure and frightened. One way I evaluate this self-confidence in a young football player is to tell him he can return to competition if he gets down in his blocking position and takes me out in the office corridor. The reactions are revealing. Some look me up and down and say, "OK, doc, I'm ready," Others simply smile, and some say "I'm not sure." When I look into their eyes, I sometimes instantly know I should say, "Hey, not this week, but come back next week and we'll reevaluate."

The fact is that you can't participate in competitive sports without aches and pains. Many of the injuries I see in my clinic are insignificant—I call them "so whats." When I've completed my examination and found no limiting injuries, I encourage the youngster to compete and not worry about the injury beyond using the proper care: ice, elastic bandages, tape, padding. Some of the "so what" injuries with which youngsters can continue to play are mild hip pointers, charley horses, shin splints, and jumper's knees. However, these are judgment calls to be made according to each individual case by the medical specialist, along with the athletes and their parents. Any permission to play should be based on clear-cut, positive medical indications, not on guesswork. If parents are anxious about the decision, I always try to resolve their concerns *before* the youngster resumes sports activity.

Despite their expertise, medical specialists cannot guarantee that an injury won't recur after return to competition. Knees are particularly vulnerable to reinjury, even after the original injury has completely healed.

In some cases, the physician may tell you that your

youngster can play with an injury, but that it may need correction after the season. An example of this was my own son Mark, who wanted to continue playing football even though he had fractured his thumb. Since there was no displacement, I gave him my "OK to go," providing that he had the fracture corrected if it became displaced. Fortunately, it stayed in place for the whole season.

An important factor in returning to competition is rehabilitation after the injury is treated. The young athlete must recover normal motion, strength, and agility before going back into action. This may require progressive therapy conducted by a registered physical therapist or certified trainer who is expert in the rehabilitation of injured athletes. All rehabilitation programs should be supervised by the physician responsible for the young athlete.

The rehabilitation process can be complicated and intensive, especially when ligaments have been surgically repaired. But even when the injury is less severe, rehabilitation must be done with great care to avoid prolonging recovery.

13

Head, Neck, and Facial Injuries

◆

◆ HEAD

Of all sports injuries, head injuries can be the least obvious and potentially the most serious. Don't let your youngster brush off a head injury by saying, "It's nothing." Let a physician decide that.

Concussion

This is a jarring injury to the head, face, or jaw resulting in a disturbance of the brain. Concussions are classified as mild or severe. Treating them can be complicated and difficult.

WHAT TO LOOK FOR:
Mild Concussion
Any or all of the following symptoms:

- Brief (if any) loss of consciousness for a few seconds to a minute
- Mild headache
- Grogginess
- Confusion
- Glassy look

196

- Brief amnesia
- Briefly disturbed balance
- Slight dizziness

Severe Concussion

Any or all of the symptoms of mild concussion (but more severe), and the following symptoms:

- Loss of awareness
- Slurred speech
- Double vision
- Nausea or vomiting
- Change of eye pupil size
- Loss of emotional control

CAUSE:

A blow to the head from an object or collision.

PREVENTION:

There is no way to prevent head injuries completely in sports, particularly contact/collision sports. But there are six important ways in which they can be *minimized*.

- A healthy athlete
- Proper equipment, including a well-fitted helmet
- Good coaching in skills
- Proper conditioning
- Good officiating
- Strengthening of neck muscles

Serious head injuries can also be reduced by disqualifying youngsters with a history of such injuries. Young athletes will often deny or forget that they had a head injury, and it is up to their parents to provide a complete history.

TREATMENT:

Generally, the trainer, coach, or physician will determine the severity of the concussion on the sidelines. Most concussions are mild and can be followed up after the game or practice, but the player should not be allowed to compete until the follow-up has been completed. Immediate care should include rest on the sidelines (either sitting or lying down), with someone in attendance to provide careful observation. Any evidence of something more serious requires an immediate trip by ambulance to a hospital for further observation. Three indications of such an emergency are: 1) unconsciousness, 2) a change in the size of the eye pupils, and 3) convulsions. Any other symptoms (see previous list)—except for the mildest complaints—call for an evaluation by a physician the same day that the injury occurred. Early recognition and diagnosis are essential in head injuries. No head injury should be taken lightly. With some injuries, called subdural or epidural hematomas, there may be a period of well-being followed in a few hours by collapse and sometimes coma.

RETURN TO COMPETITION:

The young athlete must be free of all complaints before returning to sports. *Mild* concussions may require up to a week for recovery, and the decision to return must be made by a physician. *Severe* concussions require at least four weeks, and permission to return should be given only by a specialist in head injuries.

Repeated concussions call for extra caution. When there have been three concussions—no matter how mild—specialists recommend no further competition for the season. In case of two or more *severe* concussions, returning to any contact/collision sport is not recommended.

◆ NECK

Although most neck injuries in young athletes are not serious and heal rapidly, some are devastating. Neck injuries can occur in any sport, but they occur most often in wrestling, football, and gymnastics. These injuries can also result from using a trampoline; however, trampolines have basically been removed from youth sports.

There are five types of sports injuries to the neck, ranging from minor to catastrophic:

1. Sprained neck
2. Stretch injury (also called a traction injury)
3. Ruptured disc (disc compression or herniation)
4. Cervical spine fracture without paralysis
5. Paralysis with or without spine fracture ("broken neck")

Sprained Neck

This is a kink in the neck, often called a "stiff neck" or "wry neck." It is the most common and least serious injury to the neck.

WHAT TO LOOK FOR:

Muscle spasm, stiffness, loss of motion, pain from turning or twisting the neck. However, the pain does not go down to the shoulder, arm, or back. X rays are normal.

CAUSE:

A sudden twist of the head and the neck, with or without contact with another player.

PREVENTION:

There are no specific preventive measures for avoiding neck sprains. However, they can be minimized by good conditioning with special emphasis on developing strength in the neck muscles. As with most sports injuries, neck sprains can also be kept down through good coaching, good officiating, proper equipment, and safe playing facilities. Skill in the sport is another important preventive.

TREATMENT:

A few days of rest, ice, and mild pain medication. Some trainers and physicians recommend moist heat.

RETURN TO COMPETITION:

Usually within a few days.

Traction or Stretch Injury

This is an injury to the large nerves in the neck and collarbone area, also involving the ligaments and small joints of the neck. In sports, this injury is known as a *stinger*, *burner*, or *shock*.

Don't take traction injuries lightly. If the symptoms only last a minute or two, the chances are your youngster has only suffered a mild injury. But if pain, numbness, and/ or weakness persist for more than two days, a major injury may have occurred and your youngster should not return to competition until a physician evaluates the injury.

WHAT TO LOOK FOR:

Sudden, shock-like burning, tingling, or numbness followed by a searing pain in the shoulder, upper back, or arm as far down as the hand or fingers.

CAUSE:

The head and neck are bent forcefully away from the shoulder and body, causing severe stretching. This usually occurs in lacrosse or football.

PREVENTION:

These injuries can be reduced by doing strength training exercises and wearing a cervical collar during games and practice sessions. In football, developing good skills in blocking and tackling can help.

TREATMENT:

Rest, ice, an arm sling, and pain medication if necessary. A cervical collar will give relief when the injury is severe. Expert medical care is essential if there is persistent severe pain or if the injury has recurred frequently. Even when X rays and other tests are negative, there may be a serious problem. The key indicators are how long the pain, weakness, and/or numbness last.

RETURN TO COMPETITION:

When the tingling and pain disappear quickly, little time need be lost from competition. Most traction injuries fall into this category. However, when the symptoms persist for a few days, or four or more stretch injuries occur over a period of time, the neck may become unstable. In these cases, all contact play should be stopped until a medical evaluation is made, stability tests such as X rays and electromyograms are normal, and all symptoms are absent for at least three weeks.

Ruptured Cervical Disc

When this injury occurs, the cervical discs rupture and press on the spinal cord or nerve roots. (Cervical discs are the spaces between the neck bones or vertebrae. They contain a firm, jelly-like material and act like shock absorbers and ball bearings to permit movement of the spine.)

This is a rare injury among teenage athletes. However, because it is difficult to diagnose, parents should make sure that a "stinger" or "burner" is not actually a cervical disc rupture. Don't depend on locker-room consultations with the coach, trainer, or even team physician. A visit to an orthopedic surgeon or a neurosurgeon is called for when there's any doubt. It may take sophisticated diagnostic tools, such as myelograms, electromyographs, CAT scans, or MRIs to help the doctor determine if a cervical disc rupture has occurred. Keep in mind, however, that these are only tools—

the clinical opinion of an expert physician must be the deciding factor.

WHAT TO LOOK FOR:

Severe pain in the neck or shooting pain to the shoulder and arm, stiff neck, often pain in upper back along inner margin of shoulder blade.

CAUSE:

Major impact to the head, usually with the neck bent forward and down, but sometimes upward and backward. Can also occur when the athlete uses great force to lift a heavy weight in football, wrestling, and weight lifting.

PREVENTION:

Conditioning to strengthen neck muscles can help. Other preventive factors are skill in performance, coaching, officiating, and equipment.

TREATMENT:

Relief of the pain with rest and cervical collar. In some cases, traction apparatus is required. Surgery is usually not needed by teenage athletes.

RETURN TO COMPETITION:

A minimum of six months after healing is required for return to competition.

Cervical Spine Fracture Without Paralysis

This is a fracture of a vertebra in the neck. Though a serious injury, it can heal well and should leave no permanent damage so long as the spinal cord has not been involved and the supporting bone structures are stable.

WHAT TO LOOK FOR:

Mild to severe pain in the neck.

CAUSE:

Usually a direct blow to the head or severe twisting.

PREVENTION:

Most of these injuries occur in football and can be prevented by avoiding spearing (also known as head butting, stick blocking, goring, and head blocking).

TREATMENT:

Consultation with an orthopedist or neurosurgeon is essential. Treatment usually consists of pain medication and a firm cervical collar (with four upright steel posts if the fracture is severe).

RETURN TO COMPETITION:

Definitely no more competition for that season. It's questionable whether the young athlete should ever return to contact/collision sports, because of the danger of unrecognized neck instability.

Broken Neck

This is a disruption of the spinal cord by direct compression or excessive stretching. Paralysis from a broken neck can occur without a recognized fracture or dislocation. Teenagers are more susceptible than older athletes because their bones and ligaments are still immature.

WHAT TO LOOK FOR:

Paralysis. This may be paralysis of the legs, paralysis of the legs and partial paralysis of the arms, or total paralysis of both arms and legs (*quadriplegia*).

CAUSE:

Head being driven forcefully against solid mass. Most common in recreational diving and football, but also happens in gymnastics, in wrestling, and with trampolines.

PREVENTION:

In diving: Youngsters should never dive in unknown water or shallow pools. If you have a pool, make sure it is adequately lit and guarded. Caution your teen-agers against consuming alcohol while swimming. *In football*: Warn your youngster never to use his head as a battering ram for blocking or tackling (spearing). This dangerous technique is not necessary for playing solid football.

TREATMENT:

After initial stabilization of the injury, treatment in a rehabilitation center.

◆   EYES

Serious eye injuries are rare in youth sports because the eyes are protected by a bony frame (*orbit*) that takes most of the blows. You may be apprehensive about cuts and bruises close to the eye, but they are easily treated. Only injuries to the eyeball itself and to the bony frame are potentially serious.

There are four types of sports injuries to the eyes:

1. Contusion and laceration
2. Foreign body in eye
3. Loss of vision
4. Orbital fracture

Contusion and Laceration

A contusion is a bruise and a laceration is a torn, ragged wound. These are the most common injuries about the eyes, but they are generally not serious.

WHAT TO LOOK FOR:

Possible swelling or bleeding.

CAUSE:
A blow or scrape.

PREVENTION:
Face mask or protective glasses. Skill in performance also helps.

TREATMENT:
If the injury is superficial, an ice pack and a butterfly or other type of bandage will usually suffice. Bleeding around the eye can be controlled with a gauze bandage or clean cloth under pressure. Once the bleeding is controlled, the injury should be reappraised. Some lacerations may have to be sutured at an emergency room or physician's office. Contusions or abrasions should be cleaned and dressed with a Band-Aid.

RETURN TO COMPETITION:
For mild cuts, no time need be lost. In hockey, the player sometimes returns to action after having the cut sutured in the locker room. However, severe lacerations must be completely healed before a player can resume competition. This takes from seven to ten days.

Foreign Body

Any foreign body lodged in the eye, such as a fleck of dirt, needs attention. Usually this is a nuisance condition, but if the irritation doesn't go away, it should be evaluated by an eye surgeon.

WHAT TO LOOK FOR:
Tearing, pain, and redness.

CAUSE:
Something flying into the eye.

PREVENTION:
Protective glasses can help.

TREATMENT:

Most foreign objects can be removed easily with a cotton swab and saline wash.

RETURN TO COMPETITION:

If the surface of the eye has not been seriously injured and vision is not impaired, the youngster can return to competition as soon as the foreign object has been removed.

Injury to the Eyeball

A direct injury to the eyeball is an *immediate medical emergency*.

WHAT TO LOOK FOR:

Extreme pain, loss of vision, hazy vision, double vision, change in vision colors, or obvious lacerations or abrasions of the eye.

CAUSE:

A blow to the eye from another player or a flying object such as a hockey puck or tennis ball.

PREVENTION:

The greatest need for eye protection in young sports is in ice hockey, where most serious eye injuries have occurred. Hockey injuries causing blindness have been reduced to a negligible number since helmets were made mandatory in 1978.

Sport glasses are another important source of protection against eye injuries. Every youngster entering competitive sports should undergo an eye examination by an ophthalmologist. If vision must be corrected, sport glasses with impact-resistant frames and shatterproof polycarbonate lenses are essential. Contact lenses can provide even better vision. Young athletes should always have two pairs of glasses or contact lenses.

TREATMENT:

The trainer or coach should first make sure that loss of vision is related to a direct eye injury rather than a head injury. Then a dry, sterile eyepatch or piece of gauze should be applied to the eye, along with soft crushed ice in a bag. After an advance telephone call, the injured youngster should be taken immediately to an emergency facility. Parents and school officials should be notified.

RETURN TO COMPETITION:

When the eye is totally healed, an ophthalmologist should approve return to competition, with the use of protective eye equipment.

Orbital Fracture

This is a fracture of the bony frame around the eye. All orbital fractures are serious and require expert medical treatment.

WHAT TO LOOK FOR:

Severe pain, with possible double vision and other vision problems. May be accompanied by cuts, abrasions, bleeding, and black-and-blue marks.

CAUSE:

A sharp blow to the orbital structure, usually by a punch, puck, stick, or hard ball.

PREVENTION:

Well-designed face masks are the best protection, along with skill in performance and good officiating that comes down hard on violent play.

TREATMENT:

Any significant injury to the area around the eye should be X-rayed to determine if a fracture has occurred. Orbital fractures should be seen by an ophthal-mologist or plastic surgeon.

RETURN TO COMPETITION:

Return should only be permitted after the physician approves and the young athlete is confident about going back to competition.

◆ TEETH

Teeth can be knocked out or damaged during contact/collision sports. However, a knocked-out tooth can be saved if reimplanted quickly.

WHAT TO LOOK FOR:

Loose or missing tooth, pain and/or bleeding.

CAUSE:

A sharp blow to the mouth.

PREVENTION:

Although a face mask and mouth guard can't prevent all teeth injuries in collision sports, they can reduce them to a minimum. The mouth guard is especially important, and you should insist that your youngster wear one in all contact/collision and limited-contact sports.

TREATMENT:

When a tooth is knocked out in one piece or is broken off just above the gum line, it should be found and wrapped carefully in a sterile dressing. Player and tooth should then be taken to a dentist immediately. A knocked-out tooth can be successfully reimplanted—a much less expensive procedure than replacing the tooth. However, if the tooth cannot be reimplanted within thirty minutes, it must be kept in a preserving fluid so that cells of the tooth do not degenerate. The ideal storage medium is a pH-balanced, buffered cell-preserving fluid, which is packaged in the Emergency Tooth Preserving System, available from Biological Rescue Products, Inc. This fluid can preserve and rejuvenate the tooth for up to twelve hours. Other fluids that can be used for shorter periods are whole milk, saliva, and sterile saline.

It is not practical to save a chip or small broken piece, but such damage can often be repaired through dental reconstruction.

RETURN TO COMPETITION:
Return should be based on approval by the dentist.

◆ FACE

Lacerations

Face lacerations are a common injury in almost all sports. They are generally of little consequence, but some can be severe.

WHAT TO LOOK FOR:
Pain, bleeding, possibly swelling.

CAUSE:
A direct blow from a ball, stick, punch, knee, foot, or head.

PREVENTION:
Face masks are a good preventive measure, as are skill in performance and restraints on violent play.

TREATMENT:
An ordinary cut can be sutured by a family doctor or emergency-room doctor. Severe, irregular lacerations should preferably be sutured by a plastic surgeon.

2

RETURN TO COMPETITION:

In day or two, but the cut should be protected if it is severe.

Facial Fracture

This can be a fracture of the nose, jaw, or cheekbone. Broken noses are common in sports and should not be considered a major injury. Fractures of the jaw and cheekbones are less frequent but more serious.

WHAT TO LOOK FOR:

Nose: Pain and deformity. *Jaw*: Pain with swelling; biting may hurt and be accompanied by a snapping sound. *Cheekbone*: Severe pain, marked swelling, sometimes deformity of the cheek.

CAUSE:

Sharp blow from stick, ball, etc.

PREVENTION:

Face masks, skill in performance, and restraints on violent play.

TREATMENT:

Fractured noses are correctable with plastic surgery. Jaw and cheekbone fractures should be treated by an oral surgeon or a plastic surgeon.

RETURN TO COMPETITION:

With nose and cheekbone fractures, young athletes can return after partial healing so long as they wear protection. However, a jaw fracture must be completely healed before return.

14

Upper-Extremity Injuries

♦

♦ SHOULDER

Shoulder injuries are among the most frequent in sports. In football, rugby, hockey, and men's lacrosse, shoulders are vulnerable because collision is an integral part of these games. The required force used in wrestling and gymnastics leads to many shoulder injuries. In baseball, swimming, and tennis, excessive use of the shoulder often causes damage. (For normal shoulder, see Illustration 1.)

Contusion (Bruise)

A contusion, or bruise, is the most common shoulder injury, and is seldom serious.

WHAT TO LOOK FOR:
Soreness, pain, swelling, and sometimes black-and-blue marks.

CAUSE:
Hard blow to the shoulder.

PREVENTION:
Properly fitted shoulder pads help, along with skillful performance of blocking, tackling, and other contact

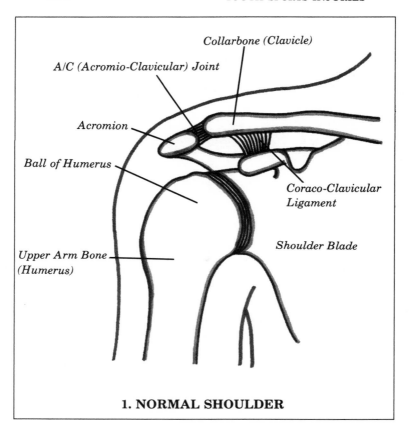

1. NORMAL SHOULDER

techniques. However, this type of injury is inevitable in contact/collision sports.

TREATMENT:

Rest and ice, followed in a day or two by light exercise to prevent stiffness.

RETURN TO COMPETITION:

In most cases, no interruption in competition is necessary. With severe cases, a few days of rest are recommended.

Sprain

The ligaments are injured by a twisting and pulling of the shoulder. This injury should be carefully evaluated to make sure it is only a sprain and not a dislocation.

WHAT TO LOOK FOR:
Soreness, pain, sometimes swelling.

CAUSE:
In addition to twisting, this injury can be caused by a direct blow.

PREVENTION:
Prevention is difficult, but conditioning and proper padding can help.

TREATMENT:
Rest, ice, and taping with a six-inch elastic bandage and/or padding.

RETURN TO COMPETITION:
Athletes can return when they have full range of shoulder motion without significant pain.

Mild Shoulder Separation (Grade 1)

When this injury occurs, the collarbone (*clavicle*) separates from the bony prominence called the *acromion* (Illustration 2). The full name is *acromio-clavicular separation*, but it is more commonly known as an *A-C separation*. The ligaments around the small joint are bruised, while the joint has a mild bump, but remains stable. This mild form of separation is no more serious than any other slight sprain.

WHAT TO LOOK FOR:
Some tenderness to the touch and pain from moving the shoulder.

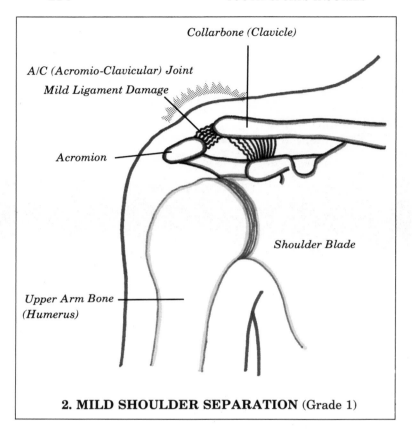

Collarbone (Clavicle)

A/C (Acromio-Clavicular) Joint

Mild Ligament Damage

Acromion

Shoulder Blade

Upper Arm Bone (Humerus)

2. MILD SHOULDER SEPARATION (Grade 1)

CAUSE:

Separation can be caused in two ways:
1. The athlete lands on the outside of the shoulder with full impact, forcing the collarbone up and out of the small joint.
2. The athlete is hit directly on the shoulder from the front, forcing the shoulder backward and pushing the joint apart.

PREVENTION:

Well-fitted shoulder pads and skill in performance can help, but these injuries are not entirely preventable in collision sports.

TREATMENT:
Rest, ice, strapping, and support with a sling.

RETURN TO COMPETITION:
Return to practice when arm can be used freely with minimal pain, usually a day or two. However, hitting and tackling should be avoided for a few more days.

Moderate Shoulder Separation (Grade 2)

This is a significant form of separation, with greater displacement of the joint. The powerful *coraco-clavicular ligament* that holds the collarbone down is stretched but still intact (Illustration 3).

WHAT TO LOOK FOR:
Greater swelling, greater pain from moving the shoulder, some weakness, and a large bump.

CAUSE:
Separation can be caused in two ways:
1. The athlete lands on the outside of the shoulder with full impact, forcing the collarbone up and out of the small joint.
2. The athlete is hit directly on the shoulder from the front, forcing the shoulder backward and pushing the joint apart.

PREVENTION:
Well-fitted shoulder pads and skill in performance can help, but these injuries are not entirely preventable in collision sports.

TREATMENT:
Rest, ice, strapping, and support with a sling.

RETURN TO COMPETITION:
Depending on the damage, it could be up to three weeks—and sometimes more—before the young ath-

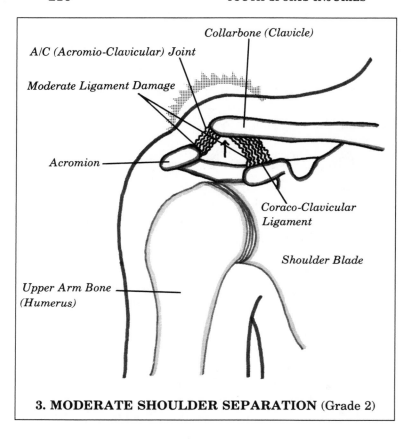

3. MODERATE SHOULDER SEPARATION (Grade 2)

lete can resume competition in a contact/collision sport. There should be no return to blocking and tackling until 1) the shoulder feels tight and solid, and 2) there is good use of the arm with minimal discomfort.

Severe Shoulder Separation (Grade 3)

The *A-C joint* is ruptured and the *coraco-clavicular ligament* completely torn (Illustration 4). This is a major injury that should be treated only by a sports medical specialist.

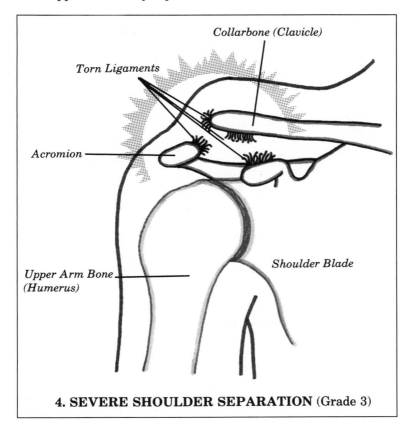

4. SEVERE SHOULDER SEPARATION (Grade 3)

WHAT TO LOOK FOR:

Severe pain, swelling, marked deformity, and inability to use shoulder.

CAUSE:

Separation can be caused in two ways:

1. The athlete lands on the outside of the shoulder with full impact, forcing the collarbone up and out of the small joint.
2. The athlete is hit directly on the shoulder from the front, forcing the shoulder backward and pushing the joint apart.

PREVENTION:

Well-fitted shoulder pads and skill in performance can help, but these injuries are not entirely preventable in collision sports.

TREATMENT:

There are two accepted methods, surgical and non-surgical. I prefer the surgical method in which a screw holds the joint in position while the ligaments heal. I have used this procedure for many years with excellent results. In the second method, a harness is placed on the shoulder and arm, with accompanying treatment of the pain and swelling. The harness is made as snug as possible and worn for four or more weeks. This is also a very acceptable approach that has been used successfully by many orthopedic surgeons.

RETURN TO COMPETITION:

A young athlete with this injury must stay out of competition for at least six to eight weeks.

Dislocation or Subluxation

Dislocation: The ball joint at the top of the large arm bone (*humerus*) comes completely out of the shoulder joint (Illustration 5). *Subluxation*: Looseness causes the ball joint to slip *partially* in and out. This looseness is usually created by a single blow. Once the supporting ligament is torn, the shoulder may dislocate or sublux repeatedly. Although this may happen infrequently, the shoulder is always in danger of further injury.

WHAT TO LOOK FOR:

If a dislocation occurs, there is severe pain, marked deformity, and total inability to use the arm. In subluxation, the pain and swelling are less severe, but it is difficult to know whether there was a dislocation that went back into position. The normal shape of the shoul-

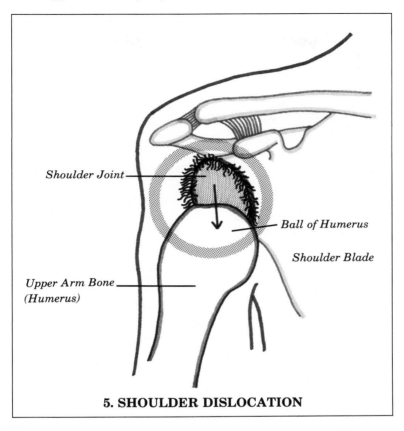

Shoulder Joint

Ball of Humerus

Shoulder Blade

Upper Arm Bone
(Humerus)

5. SHOULDER DISLOCATION

der is lost, shoulder muscles go into spasm, any movement of the arm is painful.

CAUSE:

Most often, a direct blow, usually with the arm extended. It can also occur from falling on the arm or shoulder or from a forceful throwing motion.

PREVENTION:

Preventive aids are shoulder pads, a good strengthening program, and, in football, proper blocking and tackling technique.

TREATMENT:

When a young athlete dislocates a shoulder for the first time, the treatment is rest, a sling, and no sports for four weeks. For repeated dislocations, the treatment of choice is surgical repair. Two approaches are used: (1) ligament reconstruction; (2) bone block surgery. In my opinion, the best procedure for a chronically dislocating shoulder is (1) the "Bankart operation," a surgical procedure that stabilizes the shoulder joint.

For complicated cases or recurrence after primary surgery, I go to (2) bone block surgery—also called the Bristow procedure. The choice of surgical procedures should, of course, be made by an orthopedic surgeon. Many of these surgeons prefer to use the bone block procedure first.

RETURN TO COMPETITION:

After the first dislocation, a young athlete must be out of competition for a minimum of three or four weeks, and should return only with protection from a shoulder harness. If dislocations recur no more than once a month during the season, the young athlete may return when the pain has lessened and shoulder motion is good. However, if dislocations occur more frequently, competition must be discontinued until the injury is surgically repaired.

After surgical reconstruction, a young athlete may return to the same sport in about twelve weeks. I knew a hockey player who became an All-American in college competition two years after surgery, and many youngsters who played football for years after surgery without problems. However, there is no guarantee that the shoulder will not come out again, and teenage athletes have the highest rate of such post-surgery recurrences when they return to a contact/collision sport.

Acute Rotator Cuff Injury

This sudden tear of the rotator cuff (Illustration 6) is uncommon in young athletes.

WHAT TO LOOK FOR:

Severe pain, inability to raise the arm.

CAUSE:

Occurs when the outstretched arm is wrenched in a fall.

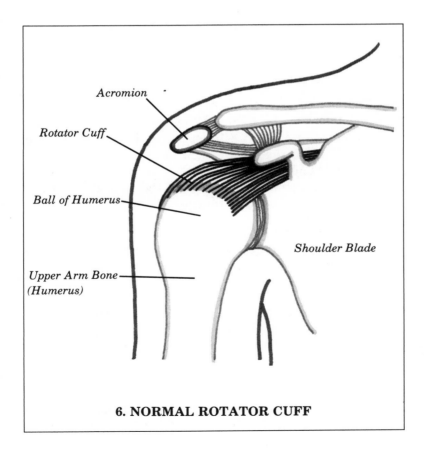

6. NORMAL ROTATOR CUFF

PREVENTION:

A difficult injury to prevent, but skill in the sport can help.

TREATMENT:

The diagnosis of this injury can be difficult, and may have to be done with a technique known as Magnetic Resonance Imaging (MRI). Another diagnostic technique that can be used is arthroscopy, in which a pencil-sized telescope is inserted into the shoulder joint to examine the injury. An arthrogram (dye test of the joint) may also help to diagnose the problem.

RETURN TO COMPETITION:

Return should only be after complete healing, which usually takes ten to twelve weeks.

Chronic Rotator Cuff Injury

This injury is a gradual fraying of the large, flat tendon that covers the top of the shoulder joint like a cuff and rotates the shoulder in a full circle. In sports activity, the cuff may catch itself under the *acromion*, which acts like a roof over the cuff and shoulder joint. This is sometimes called a "rotator cuff impingement." It is one of the most difficult and complicated of all shoulder injuries.

WHAT TO LOOK FOR:

Pain when moving the shoulder, tenderness, possible swelling.

CAUSE:

Usually caused by wear and tear from a throwing motion, such as baseball pitching. However, it can also be caused by repetitive motions in golf, tennis, and swimming, and occasionally by a single powerful blow.

PREVENTION:

The best prevention is not to permit the arm to be overused. In baseball, the number of pitches should be limited in both games and practice sessions, and the young pitcher should be taught to throw with proper form.

TREATMENT:

When this injury occurs to a young athlete, the best treatment is rest. If the condition is mild, a few days of rest will suffice. When the pain persists, three to four weeks are necessary. When baseball pitchers between twelve and nineteen have a serious, chronic condition, I may recommend an entire year off from pitching. This can preserve the youngster's chances of later returning to pitching without problems. If your youngster suffers rotator cuff pain, his coach may want him to finish out the season anyway. Don't agree to this until you consult a physician who treats young athletes. It is more important to save your young pitcher's arm so he can throw later than to save the season or the coach's job.

RETURN TO COMPETITION:

When the young athlete can throw comfortably without pain, usually after long-term rest. If this injury reoccurs, return should be based on a doctor's decision.

◆ ELBOW

Young athletes suffer few elbow injuries, but those few can be serious. Although nonstress fractures are not covered in the Home Reference Guide, the elbow fracture is being included because it is the most common serious injury to the elbow. (For a normal elbow, see Illustration 7.)

Fracture

A fracture is the most frequent serious elbow injury, occurring mainly in gymnastics, wrestling, and football.

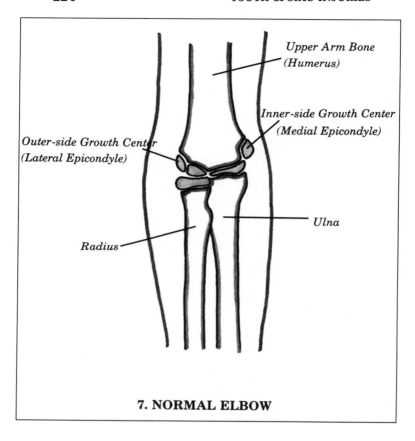

7. NORMAL ELBOW

WHAT TO LOOK FOR:

Severe pain, marked swelling, inability to move the elbow, and occasionally deformity.

CAUSE:

A fall on the outstretched hand or directly on the elbow.

PREVENTION:

Difficult to prevent.

TREATMENT:

Immediate treatment by an orthopedic specialist.

RETURN TO COMPETITION:
Only when the fracture has solidly healed and a full range of motion has returned.

Little League Elbow

This overuse injury is a strain and tearing of the muscles and ligaments about the elbow, most commonly on the inner side, although occasionally on the outer side and the front (Illustration 8). It is one of the most serious sports injuries to the elbow, most often seen in better-than-average young baseball pitchers from the age of twelve up.

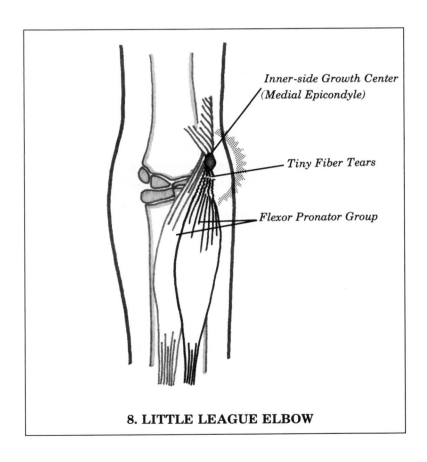

Inner-side Growth Center
(Medial Epicondyle)

Tiny Fiber Tears

Flexor Pronator Group

8. LITTLE LEAGUE ELBOW

WHAT TO LOOK FOR:

There are a number of telltale signs that the youngster's elbow may be hurting. He may hold his arm or droop his shoulder after pitches, and be sluggish and withdrawn. Although initially there may be just an ache, pain and tenderness will develop over the medial bony prominence of the elbow. With continued throwing, the elbow becomes stiff, more painful, and difficult to straighten out.

CAUSE:

This is an overuse injury that occurs when a young baseball pitcher throws too long, too hard, and too often, especially too many curve balls. Younger pitchers are particularly vulnerable from throwing curve balls before the bony development is mature. Older youths can develop Little League elbow from poor throwing habits.

PREVENTION:

Little League elbow is preventable. If you have a young pitcher—particularly one who is outstanding—keep an eye out for any signs of discomfort. If these signs are ignored, your youngster will continue to throw and get into trouble.

The first key to prevention is conditioning. The youngster should do preseason conditioning exercises and pregame warm-ups.

The second key is to limit the amount of throwing and the number of curve balls—in fact, I believe that no youngster should begin throwing curve balls until the age of fifteen.

Both the Little League and the Babe Ruth League have preventive rules that should be followed:

Ages 9–12

1. No more than four innings pitched per game
2. No more than six innings pitched per week
3. Three days rest after four innings of pitching and one day after fewer than four

Ages 13–15
1. No more than five innings pitched per day
2. No more than nine innings per week

The amount of pitching should also be limited in practice and no pitching should be allowed when the arm is hurting. The Pitching Performance Chart below is a good way to keep records.

TREATMENT:

Evaluation of Little League elbow can take some time in the sports medical clinic. Although the examination itself doesn't take long, it is essential to get a complete history of the young pitcher's throwing arm, including:

Pitching Performance Chart[1]

Date

1. Number of Innings Pitched						
2. Number of Balls Thrown						
3. "Feeling" of Arm						
4. Degree of Control						
5. Earned Runs						

[1]Taken from Allman, Fred L., Jr., M.D. *Care & Conditioning of the Pitching Arm for Little League Baseball.* Winter Park, Florida: Anna Publishing Inc., 1978.

1. How many years the youngster has been pitching
2. The pitching history in each year
3. Previous trouble
4. When the pain started
5. How many innings a week he is presently pitching
6. How hard he is throwing
7. What kinds of pitches he throws
8. How hard he throws in practice and how many days a week

After taking a history, the physician should examine the throwing arm and also the legs, shoulders, and back. Once a diagnosis is made, a recovery program should be started, with rest as the main ingredient. Several decisions must be made: First, can he pitch at all? If not, can he play another position? If the answer is no, how long will he be out of action?

The answers will depend on the severity of the injury. It's best to rely on the recommendations of a physician who regularly handles this type of problem.

RETURN TO COMPETITION:

In mild cases, pitching should be discontinued for at least two or three weeks. Other positions may be played during this period, with the exception of catcher.

With more significant injuries, a longer period of rest is required. Sometimes I recommend a whole season or even a year free from pitching. It is often difficult to get parents to accept this advice, however. Although many will say, "We'll do whatever you think is best for him, doctor," others will be less cooperative. How often I've heard, "But he's the best pitcher on the team!" or "The colleges are looking at him, you know." These are parents who push their young pitcher, often to his detriment. A long layoff from pitching at this point is absolutely necessary if he wants to pitch in later years.

Osteochondritis Dissecans

In this severe form of Little League elbow the surface of the elbow joint is damaged. Sometimes loose bodies form within the joint (Illustration 9). This condition should not be ignored, because it can leave permanent damage to the elbow joint. Continued throwing may eliminate a young picher from competition long before the big years in high school and college.

WHAT TO LOOK FOR:

Pain with and without motion, stiffness, occasional grinding or snapping sound.

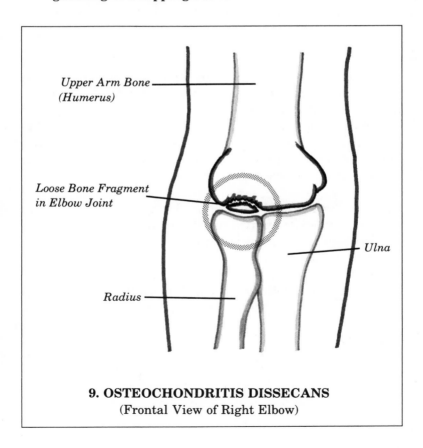

Upper Arm Bone
(Humerus)

Loose Bone Fragment
in Elbow Joint

Ulna

Radius

9. OSTEOCHONDRITIS DISSECANS
(Frontal View of Right Elbow)

CAUSE:
Excessive use of the elbow in throwing, and sometimes in gymnastics.

PREVENTION:
Control excessive throwing.

TREATMENT:
Rest from throwing and exercise. In serious cases, surgery may be required.

RETURN TO COMPETITION:
The condition must be completely resolved before competition can resume. This may take a year or more.

Tennis Elbow

This is a form of overuse tendinitis, usually on the outside of the elbow. Tennis elbow is unusual in players under nineteen, but now that some are playing all year long on professional and amateur circuits, the condition may become more common. However, it is not as serious as Little League elbow, because it is a self-limiting condition that heals well when given the opportunity.

WHAT TO LOOK FOR:
Pain when gripping a tennis racket or other object and tenderness over the prominent bone of the elbow.

CAUSE:
Excessive repetitive use of the elbow in hitting a tennis ball.

PREVENTION:
Good conditioning can help, in addition to expert coaching to correct a faulty stroke or grip.

TREATMENT:
Rest, ice, compression.

RETURN TO COMPETITION:

With mild tennis elbow, a youngster can continue to play through the season. If the condition is more severe, it should be treated by a physician before return to competition.

Traumatic Olecranon Bursitis

A large collection of fluid in a sac in the back of the elbow (Illustrations 10 and 11), this condition is of little consequence and easily treated despite its dramatic sounding name.

WHAT TO LOOK FOR:

Pain, swelling, and redness.

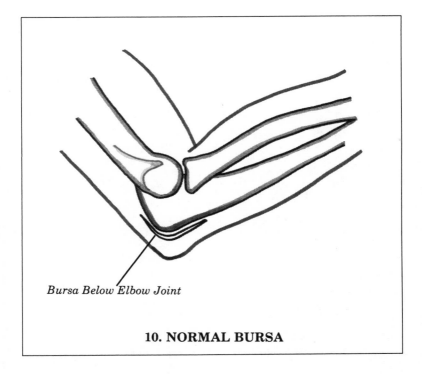

Bursa Below Elbow Joint

10. NORMAL BURSA

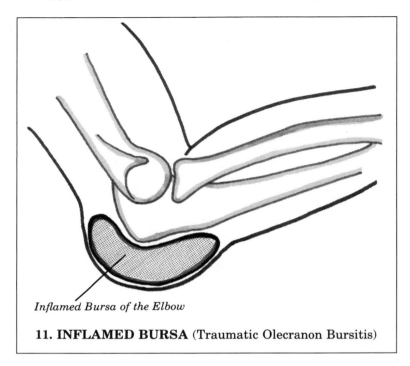

Inflamed Bursa of the Elbow

11. INFLAMED BURSA (Traumatic Olecranon Bursitis)

CAUSE:
Usually a fall on the elbow (such as when a football quarterback is sacked).

PREVENTION:
Elbow pads can help.

TREATMENT:
Rest, ice, compression, and elevation (RICE). When the injury is severe, draining the fluid with a needle can relieve it.

RETURN TO COMPETITION:
In most cases, competition need not be interrupted.

Myositis Ossificans

This is bleeding that forms a bony mass of calcium in the arm above the elbow. An uncommon condition that usually occurs in football linemen.

WHAT TO LOOK FOR:
Pain, swelling, restricted elbow motion, and sometimes stiffness in the elbow joint.

CAUSE:
Repeated blows to the arm above the elbow.

PREVENTION:
Arm pads can provide some protection, but this injury is difficult to avoid when there is hard hitting.

TREATMENT:
Rest, ice, compression, and elevation. Surgery is rarely required.

RETURN TO COMPETITION:
Athlete need not interrupt competition, but the condition should be corrected after the season.

◆ WRIST

Navicular Fracture

This is a fracture of the *navicular* bone—sometimes called the *scaphoid* bone—in the wrist (Illustration 12). Unless there is severe pain, this injury often goes unreported and unrecognized for many months after it has occurred. For example, it might happen during the football season, but nothing is done until the young athlete picks up a baseball bat in the spring and finds it too painful to hit the ball. The long-term consequences of an unhealed navicular frac-

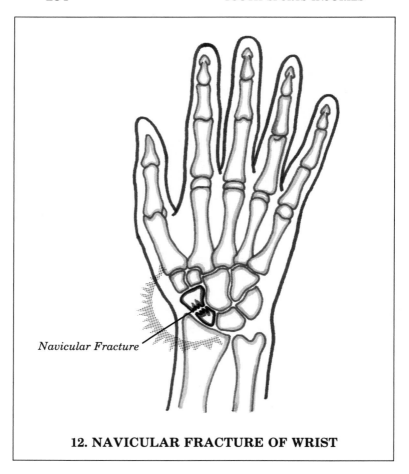

Navicular Fracture

12. NAVICULAR FRACTURE OF WRIST

ture are a disabling, painful arthritis of the wrist. That is why a "sprained" wrist should never be taken lightly.

WHAT TO LOOK FOR:

Usually appears to be a simple sprained wrist, with pain, stiffness, tenderness, or sometimes just slight soreness. But, as pointed out earlier, a "sprained wrist" should always be considered a navicular fracture until proved otherwise.

CAUSE:

A fall on the outstretched hand.

PREVENTION:

No preventive measures.

TREATMENT:

Immediate treatment is rest, ice, and compression. Every injured wrist should be X-rayed within a day or two after the injury occurs. But because the first X ray may not reveal a fracture, *it is absolutely essential to take another X ray ten to fourteen days after the first one.* (Meanwhile, the wrist should be kept in a cast or rigid splint.) If there is a fracture, it should be clearly seen in the second X ray. If there's any doubt, a bone scan will confirm the diagnosis.

When a navicular fracture is diagnosed, the treatment is a cast going from above the elbow to the tip of the thumb. Most fractures heal within six to eight weeks, but some may require six months or more—and a lot of patience.

What if the navicular fracture is discovered months after it occurred? I believe the better procedure is to treat the fracture with a long-arm cast—and resort to bone graft surgery only if this fails. However, some surgeons may recommend immediate surgery.

RETURN TO COMPETITION:

Only after solid healing of the fracture. Although some young athletes opt to continue playing with a cast, this is risky and not recommended.

Broken Wrist

This fracture of the two forearm bones—the *radius* and the *ulna*—at the wrist is probably the most common sports injury to the wrist, but young bones have a remarkable ability to heal well.

WHAT TO LOOK FOR:
Pain and deformity.

CAUSE:
A fall.

PREVENTION:
No preventive measures.

TREATMENT:
Keep in cast until healed.

RETURN TO COMPETITION:
Only after solid healing.

Tendinitis

The tendons that move the joint become inflamed. This overuse injury heals well with proper treatment.

WHAT TO LOOK FOR:
Wrist pain, with swelling and local tenderness.

CAUSE:
Repetitious wrist movement in archery, gymnastics, baseball, bowling, and any other sport that requires constant wrist or hand movement.

PREVENTION:
Good conditioning and proper skill in execution.

TREATMENT:
Rest, ice, compression, elevation, splinting.

RETURN TO COMPETITION:
No interruption is necessary if the pain permits.

◆ HAND

The most common injuries in sports are to the hand. Although most are minor, they should not be taken lightly, because the more serious injuries are difficult to spot without thorough diagnosis. A simple "finger sprain" may turn out to be a complicated fracture-dislocation. Rule one is to have all hand injuries examined by a physician. Rule two is always to have an X ray taken.

Contusion (Bruise)

Contusions usually occur to the back of the hand or the knuckles. Most are of no consequence, but always take an X ray to make sure.

WHAT TO LOOK FOR:

Bump, swelling, black-and-blue mark, tenderness to the touch, some pain. If this is simply a bruise, there should be no clicking or snapping, no feeling of the bones moving and crunching, and no weakness in the hand.

CAUSE:

A direct blow to the hand.

PREVENTION:

No preventive measures, except in certain sports such as hockey and lacrosse where gloves are required.

TREATMENT:

If the X rays prove negative and hand grip and motion are normal, the injury needs no more treatment than the application of ice and perhaps an elastic bandage with a felt pad for competition.

RETURN TO COMPETITION:

Competition need not be interrupted.

Knuckle Fracture

Although there are several types of hand fractures, the most common is a depressed knuckle fracture, sometimes known as a "punch" or "boxer's" fracture (Illustration 13). With proper treatment it heals quickly.

WHAT TO LOOK FOR:
Painful to use hand, swelling, a "dropped knuckle" (one knuckle lower than the others).

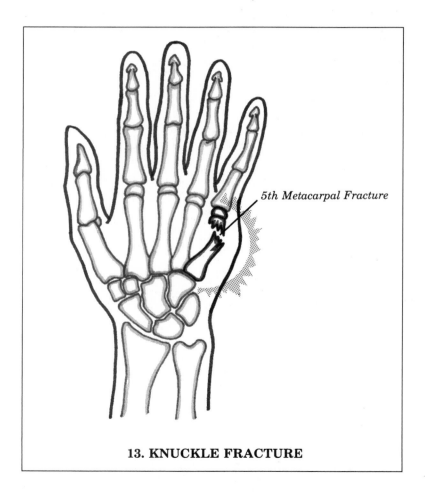

5th Metacarpal Fracture

13. KNUCKLE FRACTURE

CAUSE:

A sharp blow by or to the hand from a punch, stick, helmet, etc.

PREVENTION:

Avoid punching—which is a rules violation in all sports except boxing. Protective gloves can also help.

TREATMENT:

Expert care by a qualified physician is essential.

RETURN TO COMPETITION:

Return after solid healing, usually three to six weeks. Some young athletes return sooner, but the result can be a poorly healed bone.

Rupture of Thumb Ligament

This is a rupture of the ligament at the base of the thumb (Illustration 14). A bone chip may be torn away with

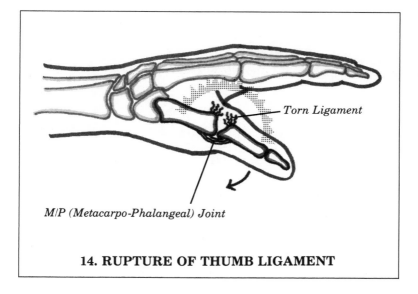

Torn Ligament

M/P (Metacarpo-Phalangeal) Joint

14. RUPTURE OF THUMB LIGAMENT

the ligament. Because they can be disabling, ligament injuries to the thumb must be given very careful treatment.

WHAT TO LOOK FOR:

Pain, swelling at the base of the thumb, looseness, and inability to pick up anything.

CAUSE:

The thumb is bent or twisted too far. This injury is common in skiing because the thumb can get caught in the ski pole strap during a fall.

PREVENTION:

In skiing, break-away ski poles can help to prevent this injury.

TREATMENT:

A cast should be applied. In some cases, surgery may be necessary. Because this apparently simple sprain may leave the thumb disabled, a ligament reconstruction may be required at a later date.

RETURN TO COMPETITION:

After the injury has healed, usually about six weeks. Sometimes the young athlete chooses to play with the injury and have the ligament reconstructed later. However, this is a risky option that I don't recommend.

Fracture of the Thumb

Most frequently, this is a fracture just above the joint at the base of the thumb. Proper medical care will prevent any permanent deformity from this injury.

WHAT TO LOOK FOR:

Pain, swelling, and inability to use the thumb.

CAUSE:

The bone is broken from a punch or being twisted too far back.

PREVENTION:

No preventive measures.

TREATMENT:

If the joint is not involved, the thumb need only be protected with a splint or small cast. When the joint itself is involved, surgical repair may be necessary.

RETURN TO COMPETITION:

With the less serious form of the injury, the young athlete can continue to play. However, a word of warning: If the fracture should displace, it then must be set by an orthopedic surgeon.

Finger Sprain

This is an injury to the ligaments that hold the finger joints together. There may be a small chip on the lower border or either side of the joint, indicating that a ligament was ruptured from the base of the joint, taking a small piece of bone with it. Such chips may get caught in the joint, creating a potentially serious problem. Finger sprains can have long-lasting effects. For example, sprained fingers frequently develop a "frustrated callus": an excessive amount of hard tissue around the joint. This is nature's way of protecting the finger from further injury. In some cases, particularly when the middle or ring finger has been sprained, the abnormal thickness may last for many years. An injury to the joint of the little finger can leave the joint stiff, no matter how good the care.

If your youngster has a finger sprain, don't try to play doctor. It is vital to get expert medical attention.

WHAT TO LOOK FOR:

Swelling, pain, and stiffness, sometimes severe.

CAUSE:

Wrenching or twisting the finger. This injury can occur in almost any sport.

PREVENTION:
No preventive measures.

TREATMENT:
Initial treatment is rest, ice, and compression. Like other finger injuries, finger sprains should always be treated by a physician.

RETURN TO COMPETITION:
Even when well cared for, finger sprains can take weeks or months to recover, so patience is required. However, in many cases, a young athlete may continue to play with this injury as long as the injured finger is taped to an adjacent finger ("buddy" taping).

Mallet Finger

The tendon at the top of the last finger joint is torn. Sometimes a fragment of bone is broken off with the tendon—if a large fragment, the joint may be displaced or dislocated. This is a classic injury seen most often in baseball, but also in basketball, football, or any sport where the finger can get jammed. It can leave a minor disability of the affected finger.

WHAT TO LOOK FOR:
The tip of the finger droops down and cannot be straightened.

CAUSE:
Usually happens when a ball hits the finger tip, but also can occur when the finger strikes a hard surface such as the ground or a helmet.

PREVENTION:
No preventive measures except skill in ball handling.

TREATMENT:
I recommend that the finger be splinted for four weeks with the tip out straight or bent upward. (The splint

and the finger may get a bit smelly, but the splint should not be removed until the end of the period.) Although this is the best treatment available, it may still leave minor disability—the finger may have a bump and not completely straighten out. Some hand surgeons recommend surgery for this injury, but I do not believe that this will produce any better results than splinting, and it's certainly far more costly.

RETURN TO COMPETITION:
A young athlete can continue to play with this injury, but should wear a padded splint.

Finger Fracture

The finger bone is fractured (Illustration 15). This common injury, which occurs in all sports, can be serious if not properly treated.

WHAT TO LOOK FOR:
Pain, deformity, and inability to use the finger.

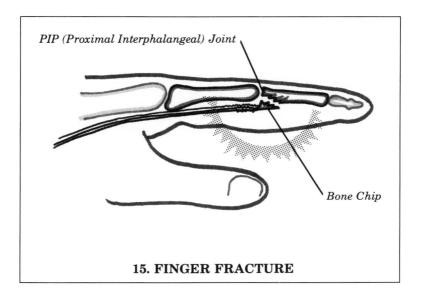

PIP (Proximal Interphalangeal) Joint

Bone Chip

15. FINGER FRACTURE

CAUSE:

Twisting the finger or receiving a direct blow to the finger.

PREVENTION:

No preventive measures, but good skills can reduce the chances of this injury.

TREATMENT:

The fractured bone should be aligned properly so that one finger does not cross over another.

RETURN TO COMPETITION:

The fracture should be completely healed before return to competition. Some young athletes may choose to play with finger fractures, but their parents should understand that this is risky.

Crushed Fingertip

The fingertip is crushed, causing a collection of blood under the nail called a *subungual hematoma*. There may be a chip fracture as well. This is a painful but insignificant injury.

WHAT TO LOOK FOR:

Severe pain, swelling, and discoloration.

CAUSE:

Fingernail may be stepped on or hit by a stick, baseball, etc.

PREVENTION:

No preventive measures.

TREATMENT:

To release the blood, a hole is made in the fingernail with a tiny drill similar to a dentist's drill. Sounds excruciating, but it's actually painless.

RETURN TO COMPETITION:
No loss of playing time is necessary in most cases.

Ruptured Tendon

A tendon that bends the fingertip is torn from the bone. A rare injury, but it has happened often enough in my experience to alert parents to its possibility.

WHAT TO LOOK FOR:
Little pain, but the muscle that bends the finger won't work.

CAUSE:
Happens in football when a player grabs for a jersey or a shoulder pad and catches the tip of a finger. For this reason, the injury is sometimes called a "jersey finger."

PREVENTION:
No preventive measures.

TREATMENT:
Surgical repair is the only choice, but it can be delayed until after the season.

RETURN TO COMPETITION:
I recommend return only after complete healing, usually ten to twelve weeks. However, a young athlete may choose to complete the season and have the injury repaired later.

15

Trunk, Abdominal, and Pelvic Injuries

◆

◆ CHEST

Serious chest injuries are uncommon among young athletes.

Getting the Wind Knocked Out

This inability to catch the breath after a severe blow to the chest or *solar plexus* is an inevitable experience for any player in contact/collision sports. Although it can be briefly traumatic, it is of no real significance.

WHAT TO LOOK FOR:
See above.

CAUSE:
Severe blow to the chest or *solar plexus*.

PREVENTION:
No preventive measures.

TREATMENT:
Treatment is simple: Give the player room to breathe and make sure there is no other injury. After a few

246

uncomfortable moments, the athlete will recover and be able to resume play. *One caution*: When asthmatic athletes get the wind knocked out, they may need more sideline care, such as a medicated inhaler.

RETURN TO COMPETITION:
As noted, as soon as the player can breathe comfortably again—usually in a few minutes.

Chest Contusion

In the past few years, several young athletes between the ages of eleven and thirteen have died after being hit on the chest-plate by a baseball or hockey puck. Why this happens is still not known.

WHAT TO LOOK FOR:
Sudden collapse of a young athlete after being struck on the chest.

CAUSE:
A blow to the chest.

PREVENTION:
A chest protector or vest can be worn at bat and on the ice. Some youth baseball leagues are using a softer ball to prevent such injuries.

TREATMENT:
Immediate CRP (cardiopulmonary resuscitation) by emergency medical technicians.

Sternoclavicular Sprain

This is an injury to the small joint located high in the chest where the collarbone joins the chest-plate. When this happens, it may be distressing to your young athlete and you, but it is usually a mild injury that heals without any major disability—although it may leave a permanent lump.

WHAT TO LOOK FOR:

The collarbone may be pushed upward and bulge at the base of the neck.

CAUSE:

A fall on the shoulder or direct blow to the upper chest.

PREVENTION:

No preventive measures.

TREATMENT:

I recommend leaving it alone. In most cases, attempting to put the collarbone back in place is a waste of time, since it will simply displace again. Operating on this joint is hazardous and generally unsuccessful.

RETURN TO COMPETITION:

When pain and tenderness are gone and the shoulder has full motion.

Costo-Chondral Sprain

An injury to the small, soft joint where the rib meets the chest-plate. Although it takes six to eight weeks to heal, this is basically a nuisance injury.

WHAT TO LOOK FOR:

Tenderness, swelling, and pain when taking a deep breath.

CAUSE:

Usually occurs in wrestling when the chest is squeezed or the athlete is thrown hard to the mat. This injury can occur in football as well.

PREVENTION:

No preventive measures.

TREATMENT:

Immediate treatment is rest, ice, and compression. The injury should then be checked by a physician to make sure it is not something more serious.

RETURN TO COMPETITION:

Usually it is safe for the wrestler to continue competing, depending on the severity of the pain.

Rib Fracture

The fracture of one or more ribs is usually of little consequence, but care should be taken with multiple fractures.

WHAT TO LOOK FOR:

It is painful to breathe and move, and the ribs are tender to the touch.

CAUSE:

Can be caused by a fall on the chest, a hard blow to the rib cage, or severe pressure on the ribs. It's most common in football from being tackled, but it can also occur in wrestling from being squeezed or thrown to the mat.

PREVENTION:

Rib pads in football and lacrosse can help, but there are no sure-fire preventive measures.

TREATMENT:

If fewer than three ribs are fractured, the basic treatment is support from a rib belt. Healing will take six weeks to the day (this is one of the few recovery times that can be predicted so precisely), and the young athlete will have to tolerate some pain. If more than three ribs are involved, the athlete should be observed carefully by a physician, because the lungs may also have been injured. When any rib is fractured in the lower left side, the injury should be diagnosed thoroughly to make sure the spleen has not been ruptured as well (see next section on ruptured spleen).

RETURN TO COMPETITION:

When one rib is broken, pain is the only limiting factor in returning to competition. With multiple rib fractures, the young athlete must be followed carefully by a physician to be sure no complications such as pleurisy occur, and return to competition should be permitted only when X rays show that the ribs have healed.

◆   ABDOMEN

Abdominal injuries are usually caused by blows to the stomach or *solar plexus*. Bruises or stretched stomach muscles are rarely of any significance and heal quickly without medical attention. The most serious stomach injuries are those that damage internal organs, especially the spleen and the kidney.

Ruptured Spleen

The spleen is a soft, lemon-sized organ located in the upper left side of the abdomen under the ribs (Illustration 16). Its function is to produce blood cells and aid the body's immune system. A ruptured spleen is the most serious sports injury to the abdomen, and should never be taken lightly.

WHAT TO LOOK FOR:

The signs of a ruptured spleen are 1) sudden pallor, 2) fainting, 3) coldness and clamminess to the touch, 4) very rapid pulse, 5) pain in the left side, and 6) lowered blood pressure. When these symptoms occur, urgent emergency procedures are imperative. If not dealt with immediately, the ruptured spleen bleeds into the abdomen, sometimes causing death.

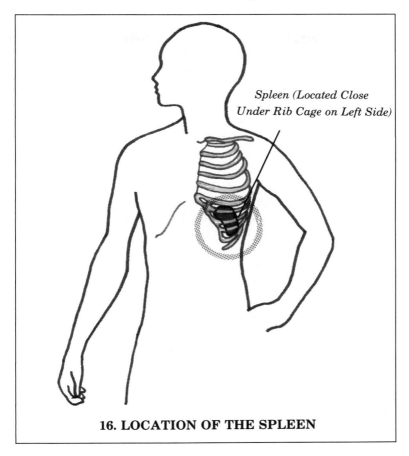

Spleen (Located Close Under Rib Cage on Left Side)

16. LOCATION OF THE SPLEEN

CAUSE:

Usually caused by a severe blow to the left side of the chest or abdomen. The greatest danger is that the player's spleen may be swollen from an unrecognized case of *infectious mononucleosis* so that it is easily ruptured.

PREVENTION:

Conditioning is one answer—the young athlete in contact/collision sports must undergo abdominal muscle toning and strengthening to be able to withstand the blows that are part of the sport. In addition, any player diagnosed with *infectious mononucleosis* must not be permitted to play in contact/collision sports until the condition has been resolved and test results are normal.

TREATMENT:

This is a red-flag emergency injury, and immediate measures must be taken to avert a tragedy. All trainers and physicians on the sidelines must be alert to the possibility of this injury and be able to recognize the symptoms. Here's where good injury-care planning is important, so that someone trained in emergency care is always on the scene and immediate transportation to a hospital is available.

RETURN TO COMPETITION:

After complete recovery—which can be ten or more weeks if *mononucleosis* is involved.

Kidney Injury

A bruise to the kidney is usually not a serious injury, and young athletes may not even report it unless the pain is severe. But parents and personnel supervising contact/collision sports such as football, rugby, and lacrosse should be alert to the possibility of a serious kidney injury.

WHAT TO LOOK FOR:

If it is mild, there will be a slight backache and some discoloration of the urine. If it is severe, there will be pain in the side, back, or flank, and the urine will turn a rusty or blood-red color. Young athletes in contact/collision sports should be instructed to report any change in the color of their urine, so that this injury will not go undiscovered.

CAUSE:

A blow to the abdomen, side, or midback.

PREVENTION:

Toning and strengthening of the stomach muscles is a good preventive measure.

TREATMENT:

In mild cases, rest until the pain is gone and the urine is clear. In severe cases, a urologist should take special tests to determine the extent of the injury, but rest is still the most common treatment, with surgery rarely needed.

RETURN TO COMPETITION:

Not until the urologist determines that the kidney has healed.

◆ BACK

It's amazing how many youngsters in sports have back pain. The trouble is, they usually report it only when questioned. In the locker room, the trainer or coach may be unaware of it. At home, you may never realize your youngster is having back pain or how severe it might be.

Back problems are frequently found in football, where power and force are placed on the young back while it is in awkward positions, and in gymnastics, where there is excessive stretching and angulation. Other athletic activities susceptible to back disorders are cross-country running, wrestling, weight lifting, basketball, diving, field hockey, ice skating, and ballet (see *Spondylolisthesis*, page 259).

Back Sprain

This is a stretching and straining that involves the muscles and ligaments in the youngster's lower back. Simple back sprains are no different from ankle sprains and will heal just as well if treated properly, but in more complicated cases, specialized care is essential.

WHAT TO LOOK FOR:

Since youngsters will often say nothing about their back sprains, it's important to recognize the symptoms. Look for:

- Expression of discomfort while standing or walking
- Pain when coughing and sneezing
- Difficulty in bending over to tie shoes
- Difficulty in getting in and out of a car
- Difficulty in sitting

CAUSE:

Most commonly caused by the back being forcefully bent backward. Another cause is overstretching. I find that coaches sometimes push their young athletes to do more stretching than is good for them. This weakens the ligaments and small joints in the back, making them vulnerable to injury. In a few cases, overstretching can lead to significant back pain, chronic back disorders, and even injury to the disc.

PREVENTION:

Trainers and coaches should recognize that their teams are made up of individual bodies of all sizes and shapes. Stretching programs should be geared to the individual athlete, rather than conditioning every youngster at the same force and pace.

TREATMENT:

The prescription is simple: Lie down as much as possible. Follow these guidelines at home:

1. Use a hard mattress. If none is available, put a ¾-inch plywood board under your youngster's regular mattress.
2. To control pain, your youngster should lie down in bed, on a couch, or on the floor, with a large pillow under the knees or the knees flexed—this relieves the ligament strain in the lower back. This should take care of most simple backaches, but the youngster must allow sufficient time for

the healing process. (It's not easy to confine an active teen-ager, but if you don't insist, the back problem could become serious.)

3. Your youngster should do orthopedic stretching exercises designed to help sprained backs (these are known as Williams exercises after the doctor who developed them).

4. Although the youngster may attend classes, sitting should be avoided at other times.

This treatment should heal a simple back sprain. However, if the problem persists for a week, your youngster should visit a physician. To determine the severity of the problem, the physician may order an MRI or CAT scan or send your youngster to a neurosurgeon or orthopedist for a consultation.

RETURN TO COMPETITION:
Only a physician should make this judgment call.

Disc Injury

Between the bones in the back are discs with a fibrous outer layer surrounding a jelly-like substance. They have a cushioning effect that permits back movement. Sports activity can damage these discs, causing pressure on the sciatic nerve (Illustration 17). This injury is known variously as slipped, herniated, or ruptured discs. It is likely to eliminate the young athlete from the sport in which it occurred, and perhaps from other sports as well.

WHAT TO LOOK FOR:
Severe spasm and pain, along with back stiffness. A pain radiating to the buttocks, hip, thigh, leg, or foot indicates involvement of the sciatic nerve—a large nerve with branches from the buttocks to the legs. Pain, numbness, or tingling in the leg or foot also means sciatic nerve compression. These are red-flag symptoms that signal a major problem.

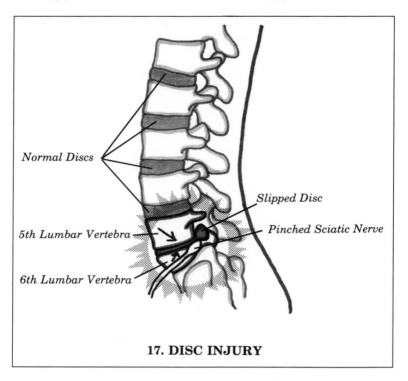

Normal Discs

Slipped Disc

5th Lumbar Vertebra

Pinched Sciatic Nerve

6th Lumbar Vertebra

17. DISC INJURY

CAUSE:
Too much force placed on the back.

PREVENTION:
Strengthening, conditioning, controlled stretching, and skill in performance.

TREATMENT:
Same as for back sprain, but should be treated only by a neurosurgeon or orthopedic surgeon.

RETURN TO COMPETITION:
Six months after all symptoms are absent.

Lower Spine Fracture (Transverse Process)

A stress fracture in which the horizontal bony struts that support the back muscles snap and break (Illustration 18), this is a painful but not serious injury. However, it is important to make sure there has been no accompanying injury to the kidney.

WHAT TO LOOK FOR:
Severe back pain, with marked spasm of the muscles.

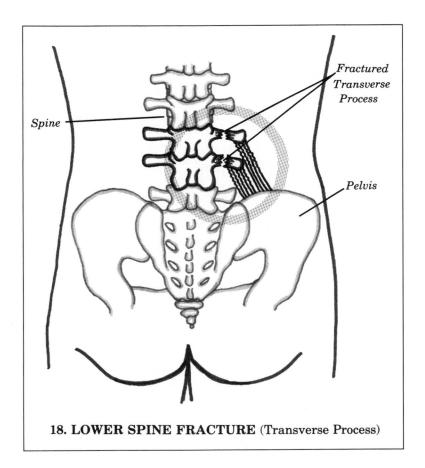

18. LOWER SPINE FRACTURE (Transverse Process)

CAUSE:
Usually occurs in football from forcefully using the back muscles or severely twisting the back.

PREVENTION:
No preventive measures.

TREATMENT:
Rest until free of pain.

RETURN TO COMPETITION:
After the pain subsides and normal motion returns—usually four weeks.

Lower Spine Fracture (Compression)

A fracture of one or more back bones resulting from compression, it heals well with no residual disability.

WHAT TO LOOK FOR:
Severe, disabling back pain.

CAUSE:
These fractures occur when the lower back is acutely flexed with great force. Most common in gymnastics, football, and tobogganing.

PREVENTION:
Strength training and skill in performance can reduce the possibility of this injury, but can't prevent it completely.

TREATMENT:
Rest is the primary treatment. After the pain has subsided and the young athlete can move about, a brace should be worn. It is most important to avoid reinjury during the healing process.

RETURN TO COMPETITION:
From three to six months, depending on the severity of the injury.

Spondylolisthesis

This is a defect of the bones that support the frame of the vertebrae (back bones), which protect the spinal cord (Illustration 19). Instead of the normal solid struts of bone, these supports are made up of soft, fibrous ligaments. I be-

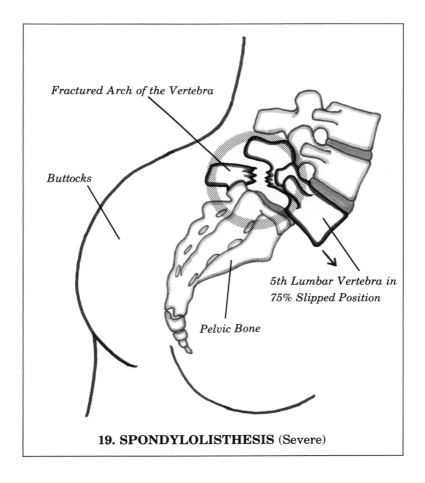

Fractured Arch of the Vertebra

Buttocks

5th Lumbar Vertebra in 75% Slipped Position

Pelvic Bone

19. SPONDYLOLISTHESIS (Severe)

lieve that a youngster with this back condition should be steered away from gymnastics and ballet. Decisions on such sports as football and wrestling should be made individually, based on clinical findings (rather than X rays), the medical history, and the amount of pain involved. I have approved participation in football, soccer, and basketball when the history does not indicate a serious problem and the youngster can bend freely without pain.

WHAT TO LOOK FOR:

Spinal instability and weakness. In some cases, when the vertebrae actually slip forward, there can be disabling pain.

CAUSE:

Generally considered to be a congenital defect. However, there is also clinical evidence that it can be caused by a fracture of the bony supports, most commonly in young gymnasts who flex and extend the spine repeatedly under force.

PREVENTION:

There is no way to prevent the congenital condition. However, making sure that youngsters with this condition do not compete in sports that involve excessive back flexing can reduce the chances of worsening the condition.

TREATMENT:

Mild cases are treated as a back sprain. More severe cases may require a back brace, and the most complicated cases may need surgery.

RETURN TO COMPETITION:

In mild cases, the young athlete may return when the pain is gone—usually in about three weeks. In more severe cases, sports competition may have to be permanently discontinued.

◆ **MALE GENITALS**

Impact Injury

This is an injury from a direct blow to the genitals—rarely serious, but one of the greatest pains in sports!

WHAT TO LOOK FOR:
Excruciating pain, which fortunately lasts only a few minutes.

CAUSE:
Direct blow to the genitals.

PREVENTION:
Jockstrap with protective cup and heavy pads.

TREATMENT:
None usually needed—however, if a severe injury occurs, ice should be applied immediately and the genitals should be examined by a physician.

RETURN TO COMPETITION:
The young athlete can return as soon as the pain subsides—normally a few minutes.

Jock Itch

An irritation of the skin in the crotch, it can sometimes develop into a fungus infection. This condition causes discomfort, but is not serious and can be easily prevented or remedied.

WHAT TO LOOK FOR:
Itching, rash.

CAUSE:
Chafing, sweating, lack of cleanliness. Very common in bicycling, but occurs in most other sports as well, especially at the beginning of a season.

PREVENTION:
Frequent showers and clean, properly fitting jockstraps and underwear.

TREATMENT:
Easily treated by washing with soap and wearing a clean, properly fitting jockstrap. An actual infection will respond to an over-the-counter antifungal medicine.

RETURN TO COMPETITION:
Unless there is excessive discomfort, the young athlete may keep competing.

◆   FEMALE GENITALS

Impact Injury

This is an injury to the genitals from a direct blow. Although female genital injuries are uncommon, they can occur in ice hockey and lacrosse, as well as in equestrian jumping from a fence fall.

WHAT TO LOOK FOR:
Severe pain.

CAUSE:
Direct blow to the genitals.

PREVENTION:
Wearing a pelvic protector.

TREATMENT:
No treatment usually is needed. The pain normally subsides in a few minutes and any swelling goes down within a few days.

RETURN TO COMPETITION:
In most cases, no interruption is necessary.

Water-Skiing Douche

This injury to the vagina is becoming more common with the growing popularity of water skiing as a competitive sport for youngsters.

WHAT TO LOOK FOR:
Painful internal and external swelling.

CAUSE:
Occurs during water skiing when water is driven into the vagina with excessive force.

PREVENTION:
Skill in performance.

TREATMENT:
This is a severe injury calling for emergency medical treatment.

RETURN TO COMPETITION:
When injury has healed, as determined by a physician.

16

Lower-Extremity Injuries

◆

Almost every action in sports requires the legs to perform with force and skill. Legs provide the speed and agility that young athletes need to compete successfully. At the same time, legs endure more stress and injury than any other part of the body. Leg complaints are seen in the doctor's office every day—some serious, some not. This section deals with injuries to all parts of the leg except the knee. Because knee injuries are the most troublesome in sports, they are discussed separately in the next chapter.

◆ HIP

Hip Pointer

This injury to the bony point of the hip (Illustrations 20 and 21) may be either a contusion or a sharp tearing of the muscle. In the injury's most severe form, a small fragment of bone may be torn away—this is called an *avulsion fracture* (Illustration 22). Hip pointers heal well without permanent effects.

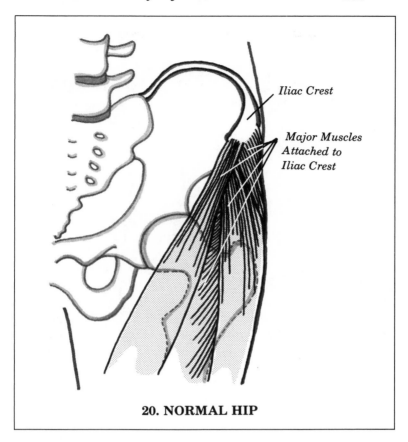

Iliac Crest

Major Muscles
Attached to
Iliac Crest

20. NORMAL HIP

WHAT TO LOOK FOR:

Local pain, sometimes severe tenderness to the touch,
inability to climb stairs, pain when walking, and at
times swelling on the side of the hipbone.

CAUSE:

A direct blow or a sudden stretching of the muscles
from such actions as making a quick turn, sprinting,
or blocking in football.

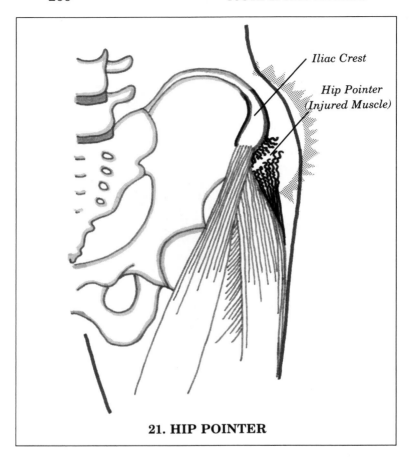

Iliac Crest

*Hip Pointer
(Injured Muscle)*

21. HIP POINTER

PREVENTION:

Wearing hip pads, conditioning, and stretching help, but this injury is not always preventable.

TREATMENT:

Usually treated with rest, ice, compression, and elevation. If there is a large tear of the muscle, crutches may be needed. A ¾-inch-thick pad in the heel of the shoe can be used to take the pressure from the front of the hip, and the hip can be strapped in a figure-eight

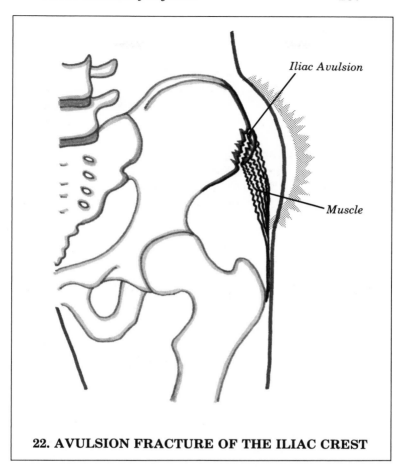

Iliac Avulsion

Muscle

22. AVULSION FRACTURE OF THE ILIAC CREST

pattern for compression and support. An avulsion fracture can take months to heal completely, but it leaves no residual disability.

RETURN TO COMPETITION:

If the hip pointer is mild, only a few days may be needed before returning to competition. A severe tear or an avulsion fracture can restrict the athlete for eight to ten weeks.

Groin Pull

A groin pull is similar to a hip pointer, except that the muscles tear from the groin rather than from the bony point of the hip. A severe groin pull can cause a small fragment to break away from the deep bone in the groin. This injury takes many weeks to heal, but leaves no residual disability.

WHAT TO LOOK FOR:

Deep pain when walking, tenderness in the groin, stiffness in the hip joint, and inability to run.

CAUSE:

Sudden force or direct blow.

PREVENTION:

Conditioning, stretching, and strength and endurance training.

TREATMENT:

Should be treated like a hip pointer with rest, ice, and a compression bandage. Crutches may be necessary. A ¾-inch-thick pad in the heel of the shoe can take pressure off the front of the hip.

RETURN TO COMPETITION:

If the pull is mild, only a few days may be needed before returning to competition. A severe tear can restrict the athlete for eight to ten weeks.

Stress Fracture in the Hip Area

This is a crack in the neck of the hipbone or the rim of the pelvis. It is also called a *silent* or *occult* fracture. This injury is a good example of why parents should not ignore aches and pains that don't go away. Proper treatment of these stress fractures is imperative.

Conditions That Simulate Hip Injuries

An apparent hip injury is not always what it seems—it can be a medical condition that affects the hip or a back condition.

Synovitis. *This is an inflammation of the hip joint with the cause usually unknown. It occurs primarily in youngsters six to ten years old, but occasionally in teenagers. When this condition is diagnosed, it should be treated by both a pediatrician and an orthopedist.*

Slipped Epiphysis. *This is an abnormal instability in the growth line at the hip joint that causes the ball of the joint to slip. The cause is unknown. It is most often seen in overweight, underdeveloped boys and girls, occasionally in a tall, lanky teenager. It is char-acterized by a persistent limp, and is a red-flag injury that calls for treatment by an orthopedist. Always keep in mind that any limp lasting more than a few days may be an* orthopedic emergency. Don't take any chances—have your youngster checked by an orthopedic surgeon.

Pain Referred to Hip. *Your youngster may have a pain in the hip, but the source could be somewhere else. It is not unusual for hip pain to be caused by a low-back disorder, such as a ruptured disc. Whenever there is persistent hip pain which does not go away in a reasonable time, these possibilities should be in-vestigated by a physician.*

WHAT TO LOOK FOR:

Pain in hip and groin while running, walking, and climbing stairs.

CAUSE:

This injury is usually caused by prolonged running during the early stages of training.

PREVENTION:

Progressive training and conditioning can reduce these injuries.

TREATMENT:

Since this injury can be difficult to diagnose, any suspicion of it must be carefully checked out. If the fracture does not show up on an X ray, the young athlete should undergo a bone scan or MRI for further diagnosis. A fracture of the femur at the hip is a red-flag injury. If not treated properly, it may not heal, and major surgery could be necessary.

RETURN TO COMPETITION:

Stress fractures take up to eight weeks to heal, and it is absolutely essential, especially with hipbone fractures, for complete healing to take place before the young athlete returns to sports.

◆ THIGH

Thigh Muscle Tear

At the front of the thigh is a large muscle (*quadriceps*) made up of four parts that work together to flex the hip and straighten the leg. When this muscle is pulled, a tear can occur, sometimes called the *quadriceps pull*. It can be a simple light catch or a complete rupture. This injury is usually mild but can be severe enough to require surgery. Early care by the trainer or physician can minimize the injury and time lost from competition.

WHAT TO LOOK FOR:

Thigh pain, swelling, a stiff knee joint, and inability to walk.

CAUSE:

Forceful use of the thigh (such as punting a football) or a direct blow to the thigh.

PREVENTION:

Properly fitted thigh pads, conditioning, strength training, and stretching.

TREATMENT:

A thigh muscle tear should be treated immediately with ice to prevent worsening of the injury. After that, the treatment is rest, time, and physical therapy for all except the most serious cases when the muscle totally ruptures. For these cases, surgical repair may be needed.

Occasionally, a small permanent dimple in the thigh may remain from the injury.

RETURN TO COMPETITION:

No time need be lost from mild injuries, but the whole season may be lost in more severe cases.

Charley Horse

A contusion of the thigh muscle, it causes bleeding inside the thigh. An ordinary charley horse is a classic sports injury of no consequence that is often not even reported by the athlete.

WHAT TO LOOK FOR:

Swelling, pain and stiffness, and possibly black-and-blue marks.

CAUSE:

A direct blow to the thigh by someone's knee, a hockey stick, a helmet, etc.

PREVENTION:

Properly fitting thigh pads, conditioning and stretching.

TREATMENT:
Rest, ice, compression, elevation, and, in some cases, crutches.

RETURN TO COMPETITION:
There may be no time lost, or a week at worst.

Myositis Ossificans

This term—meaning "bone in the muscle"—is used for massive bleeding in the thigh that causes a bony formation or ossification frequently limiting use of the thigh for from three to six weeks (Illustration 23). This is the most severe

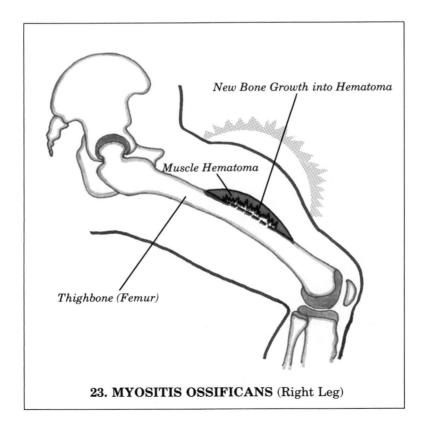

New Bone Growth into Hematoma

Muscle Hematoma

Thighbone (Femur)

23. MYOSITIS OSSIFICANS (Right Leg)

form of a charley horse, but in almost all cases, recovery is complete.

WHAT TO LOOK FOR:

The entire thigh muscle swells and there may be complete disability of the muscle. The knee also may swell, with fluid forming in the knee joint.

CAUSE:

A direct blow to the thigh.

PREVENTION:

Properly fitting thigh pads.

TREATMENT:

A massive hemorrhage should be treated as an emergency. A large, crushed-ice pack should immediately be applied to the entire muscle, and the leg should be wrapped in a compression bandage from the ankle to the hip. This should be followed by complete rest.

More moderate cases of *myositis ossificans* are often not recognized until the bony formation occurs later. In this case, the treatment is to restore the strength and motion of the thigh and knee through a professional rehabilitation program. On rare occasions, the bony mass becomes so large that it hinders use of the thigh muscle and must be removed surgically.

RETURN TO COMPETITION:

When the young athlete has recovered thigh strength, and can straighten the leg out completely and squat down comfortably.

Hamstring Tear

The hamstring muscles most commonly tear from the upper center of the muscle, but occasionally from the pelvic bone under the buttocks, and more rarely from the knee area. Hamstring tears range from mildly to severely disabling. Those with no swelling, tenderness, or black-and-blue marks could actually be lower-back disorders, especially when they occur in distance runners. I call this "silent sciatica."

WHAT TO LOOK FOR:

Disability, pain, swelling (sometimes massive), and occasionally black-and-blue marks.

CAUSE:

Hamstring pulls result from the sudden, forceful acceleration that is required in track and some field sports.

PREVENTION:

Conditioning, strength training, and stretching.

TREATMENT:

Rest, ice, compression, sometimes crutches.

RETURN TO COMPETITION:

Return ranges from after a few days to not until the next season, depending on the severity of the tear.

Hamstring Avulsion Fracture

This injury occurs when a small fragment of bone is torn with the muscles from the back of the hip under the buttocks, where the hamstrings are connected to the pelvis. A major overuse injury, it can require plenty of patience from everyone involved: the young athlete, parents, coaches, and trainers.

WHAT TO LOOK FOR:

Pain, swelling, inability to walk, tenderness under the buttocks, loss of hip motion. A large area of the thigh may turn black-and-blue after a day or two.

CAUSE:

Using the hamstring muscles with great force, such as in hurdling.

PREVENTION:
Stretching and conditioning.

TREATMENT:
Rest, ice, compression with a figure-eight bandage, and crutches when severe, followed by extensive rehabilitation.

RETURN TO COMPETITION:
For mild tears, about a week is sufficient. Extensive tears cause a lengthy disability. For example, one of the top-ranked high hurdlers in the United States suffered this injury shortly before his state finals and took a year to recover his full speed.

◆   **LOWER LEG**

Young athletes under nineteen years old suffer few serious lower-leg injuries. However, you should be aware of four types of injuries that can occur to your young athlete: contusion, shin splints, stress fracture, and anterior compartment syndrome. With the exception of stress fractures, lower-leg fractures will not be discussed here because they are routine orthopedic problems not specific to sports.

Contusion

This is a bruise of the shin. Many contusions simply cause a black-and-blue mark and some soreness, then clear up with little attention. A small percentage, however, can cause more concern. When the injury is directly over the shin bone (*tibia*), particularly just above the ankle, blood may accumulate under the lining of the bone, forming a hard mass which at first is tender and then becomes almost as hard as bone. Although this lump can be as small as a peanut, it is usually walnut-sized and occasionally larger. Despite the worry this can cause, it shrinks and eventually dissolves completely. Rarely, there may be a permanent bump under the skin. Leg bruises are common and generally nothing to worry about.

WHAT TO LOOK FOR:
Pain, swelling, and black-and-blue marks.

CAUSE:
Hard blow to the shin.

PREVENTION:
Well-fitted shin pads (these are required in field hockey).

TREATMENT:
Rest, ice, compression, and elevation.

RETURN TO COMPETITION:
No time need be lost unless the pain is excessive.

Muscle Cramp

This spasm or cramping of the muscles usually occurs in the calf but sometimes in the thigh or hamstring. It is a temporary condition of little consequence.

WHAT TO LOOK FOR:
Sudden, severe pain in the back of the calf that eases in a few minutes. The muscle may be very tender and tight or rock hard.

CAUSE:
Although the cause is not certain, loss of salt in the muscle is suspected.

PREVENTION:
Stretching and conditioning.

TREATMENT:
Treatment is usually to stretch the muscle by pulling at the ankle. Ice and massage may also help.

RETURN TO COMPETITION:

As soon as the spasm is relieved and the leg is flexible.

Shin Splints

Actually, no one is really sure just what shin splints are, beyond the fact that they cause pain in the shin from running. The injury occurs most frequently to distance runners, but also to sprinters, tennis players, and those involved in other running sports. Although not a permanent injury, it can be intensely frustrating to otherwise healthy athletes.

WHAT TO LOOK FOR:

Pain and tenderness developing along the front edge of the shin where the muscles are attached. These symptoms can show up suddenly, but usually develop gradually. Swelling and discoloration are seldom seen.

CAUSE:

This is an overuse injury similar to tennis elbow and jumper's knee. There are many different opinions as to the specific cause, including: changing training techniques, overrunning, lower-back problems, difficulty with shoes, the shape and structure of the leg, the position of the kneecap in relation to the leg, and the angle of the heel cord.

PREVENTION:

First, careful review of the training plans for the youngster before the season starts. Then, progressive workouts and training, including stretching and conditioning before running. Proper shoes and good running form are also important.

TREATMENT:

Because we lack scientific knowledge about shin splints, a wide variety of treatments has sprung up. Every trainer and sports physician seems to have a favorite cure: ice massage, strapping and taping, stretching, exercise, heel pads, different shoes, arch supports, medication, liniments, a different running form, a revised training schedule, etc. However, in my opinion, the best treatment is plain rest.

RETURN TO COMPETITION:

Return to competition is often mishandled. The youngster with shin splints is turned into a human yo-yo with an endless cycle of rest-run-pain-rest-run-pain. Eventually, youngsters going through this cycle lose their self-esteem because they're afraid people will think they're not doing their best.

Shin splints are not permanent, so returning to competition is a personal decision. If the youngsters themselves are willing to perform with some pain, let them do it—but don't let them be pushed by insistent coaches.

Anterior Compartment Syndrome

This is a devastating injury caused by a blow to the front of the lower leg. Bleeding into the leg muscles causes severe pressure that crushes the muscles and the nerves, and the major nerve to the foot becomes permanently paralyzed, resulting in a "drop foot." In this condition, the muscles can no longer lift the foot, so it drags and slaps during walking. If the condition is severe enough, a brace is required.

While rare, the anterior compartment syndrome vividly points up why a sports injury should never be taken for granted until it is accurately diagnosed. Unfortunately, even physicians can miss this injury, and the delay in treatment often leads to tragedy. The more informed that athletes, parents, coaches, and physicians are about this injury, the greater the chance of avoiding permanent damage.

WHAT TO LOOK FOR:

Pain and swelling at the front of the leg. These symptoms may be so deceptively mild at first that the youngster is not even taken to the emergency room until it's too late, because this is a red-flag injury that must be operated on immediately. Even if taken to the emergency room, the youngster may be given simple care and told to see an orthopedic surgeon later if the condition hasn't improved. But after the youngster leaves the hospital, the pain becomes excruciating and the muscles become tense and bulging, while the skin takes on a glossy sheen. By this time, it may be too late to prevent permanent damage.

CAUSE:

Usually occurs in football from a direct blow to the front of the leg. It can also occur in other collision sports such as field hockey, lacrosse, and ice hockey.

PREVENTION:

Although there is no way to prevent the initial injury, permanent damage can be prevented through immediate recognition by the trainer or physician.

TREATMENT:

If the injury is diagnosed immediately, emergency surgery can relieve the pressure and prevent permanent damage.

RETURN TO COMPETITION:

Only after complete healing. When there is permanent nerve damage, running skills and competitive sports will be limited.

Stress Fracture

This overuse injury starts out as a microscopic fracture (Illustration 24), so it is difficult to diagnose right away because it doesn't show up on X rays for ten to fourteen days. Until then, the diagnosis must be based on history and physical examination, which may be a challenging task for the physician. This is one of the simplest sports injuries,

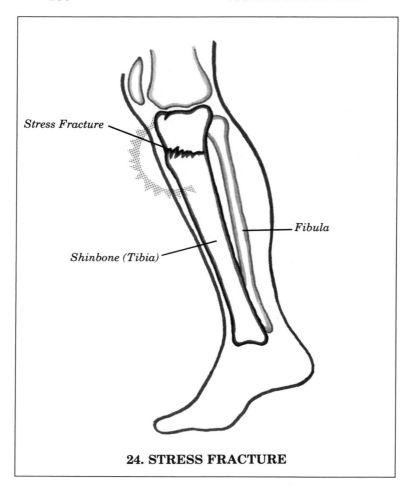

Stress Fracture

Fibula

Shinbone (Tibia)

24. STRESS FRACTURE

yet one of the most frustrating, because it means interruption of sports activity.

WHAT TO LOOK FOR:

Usually pain in the leg, shin, foot, or knee.

CAUSE:

Stress fractures are another overuse syndrome. Run too long, too hard, and too fast, and a bone may crack.

PREVENTION:

Proper training and conditioning in all sports. Excessive training should be avoided.

TREATMENT:

Every effort should be made to diagnose a stress fracture early, because the sooner an athlete stops competing the sooner it will heal. The basic treatment is rest until the fracture has healed, usually six weeks. A cast is not necessary. However, it is important to follow the fracture through a series of X rays until it has healed, because occasionally it doesn't heal. This can lead to future problems, including long-term disability and, in rare cases, the need for corrective surgery.

RETURN TO COMPETITION:

When the fracture is healed and the youngster can move and run without pain.

◆ ANKLE

Injuries to the ankle are among the most common in sports. Although most of them are not serious, it is essential to investigate every injury carefully. X rays are a must, because a "simple" sprained ankle could actually be a displaced fracture. A misdiagnosis can incapacitate a young athlete for a long time. *Example*: A great college quarterback was treated for a "sprained ankle" that turned out to be a fracture requiring surgery to repair the damage that had been done. He never played as well again.

Ankle Sprain

This is an injury to the ligaments that stabilize the ankle. There are two basic ligaments that can be damaged. On the outside of the ankle is the *lateral ligament* (Illustration 25). On the inside is the *medial ligament* (Illustration

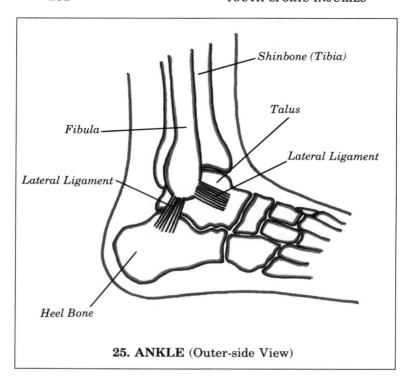

25. ANKLE (Outer-side View)

26)—also called the *deltoid*—which acts as a broad, powerful support. Most ankle sprains involve the outside, or lateral, ligaments. When the medial ligament on the inner side of the ankle is also involved, the injury is more serious. All ankle sprains should be seen as soon a possible by an orthopedist.

Ankle sprains are classified by severity:

- *Grade 1 (Mild)*: The lateral ligament is stretched but still intact. Bleeding is minimal, and there is mild pain and swelling with no instability. The young athlete may have the feeling that his or her ankle "popped."
- *Grade 2 (Moderate)*: This involves a partial rupture of the ligament, moderate bleeding, more severe pain and swelling, and inability to walk on the ankle. The medial (deltoid) ligament may be involved, but not seriously.

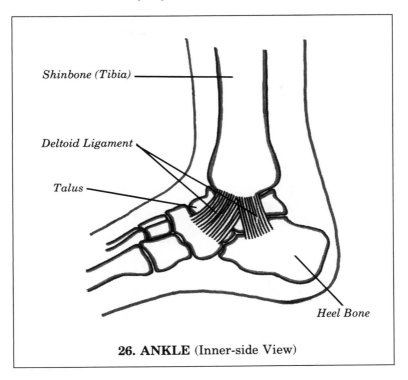

Shinbone (Tibia)

Deltoid Ligament

Talus

Heel Bone

26. ANKLE (Inner-side View)

• *Grade 3 (Severe)*: A complete tear of the lateral ligament, with severe pain, extensive bleeding, swelling, and definite involvement of the medial ligament on the inside of the ankle (Illustration 27). The injured athlete is unable to bear weight on the ankle or even put it down. There may be a feeling of complete dislocation, even though that may not have happened.

WHAT TO LOOK FOR:

In addition to the symptoms described above for the three grades of sprains, the ankle may turn black-and-blue.

CAUSE:

The foot turns sharply under the ankle.

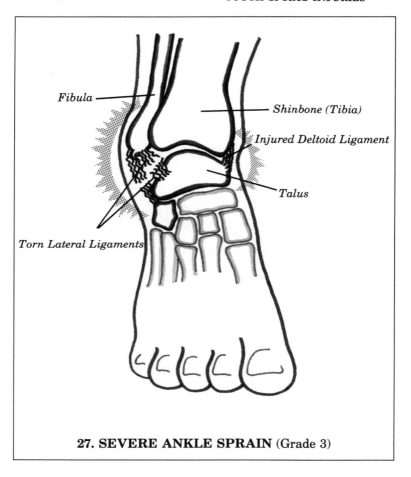

27. SEVERE ANKLE SPRAIN (Grade 3)

PREVENTION:

There is really no way to prevent a sprained ankle. Ankle wraps are used in most colleges and some high schools, but most sports medical specialists agree that these wraps are not effective enough to justify their expense.

TREATMENT:

Rest, ice, compression, and elevation. Accurate diagnosis of the ligaments involved and expert care are essential. Most important is an X ray to rule out a fracture. Then it must be decided whether an elastic bandage and crutches are adequate treatment or whether a boot cast is necessary. A recent innovative technique is to apply an air splint immediately after a sprain.

In the case of total ligament ruptures, particularly to the inside (medial) ligaments, surgery may be required—but these instances are rare. In my view, operating immediately on acute lateral ligament tears is not indicated for young people. However, lateral ligaments may become chronically unstable when not given adequate time to heal or when the ankle is repeatedly sprained. This instability can be corrected by a surgical ligament repair.

RETURN TO COMPETITION:

It is most important to avoid excess use of the ankle before the swelling and tenderness subside. The best test for return to competition is simple: The young athlete can jump up and down comfortably on the ankle. But an injured ankle must always be protected, either by taping or by an air splint—a plastic device that is wrapped around the ankle and then inflated to provide an air cushion. However, neither of these measures can guarantee that the ankle will not be reinjured.

◆ FOOT

Young athletes seldom have foot problems. Of the problems they do have, the most typical is a simple foot strain, but there are other problems that can be nagging. Even though a foot injury may seem to be minor, an X ray should always be taken because the injury could be far more serious than it appears. I know of a college football player who appeared to have simply "twisted his foot." No X rays were taken for several weeks. By that time there had been permanent damage to the foot requiring extensive surgery, and this outstanding athlete never regained his playing power. The moral is: No second-guessing with foot injuries—get an early X ray and expert opinion. (For a normal foot, see Illustration 28.)

Blister

A collection of fluid in areas of the foot subject to pressure or friction, this problem is usually seen early in the playing season.

WHAT TO LOOK FOR:
Swelling, redness, and pain that can be severe.

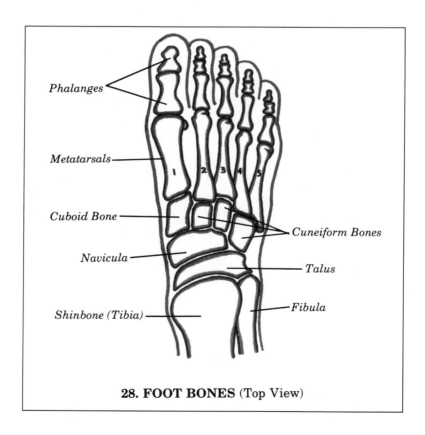

Phalanges

Metatarsals

Cuboid Bone

Cuneiform Bones

Navicula

Talus

Shinbone (Tibia)

Fibula

28. FOOT BONES (Top View)

CAUSE:

New shoes or sneakers, poorly fitted socks, or excessive running when the feet are not in good condition.

PREVENTION:

Well-fitting shoes and sneakers that are broken in gradually, properly fitting socks, foot powder, and progressive increase in the amount of running at the beginning of a season.

TREATMENT:

Keep affected area clean, correct the cause of the blister, drain the fluid if excessive, and apply a moleskin bandage.

RETURN TO COMPETITION:

When pain permits, with protection from a "doughnut" pad that fits around the blister.

Foot Strain

A stretch or partial tear of the ligaments that support the foot, this is an early-season complaint that usually only lasts for several days but sometimes for weeks. Although it's not a serious injury, the foot should be X-rayed to rule out a stress fracture or an underlying congenital problem.

WHAT TO LOOK FOR:

Pain in the instep, arch, or ball of the foot (Illustration 29).

CAUSE:

Overuse after a period of inactivity is the usual cause. For example, an athlete running in the spring after laying off all winter is vulnerable to foot strain. It also can be caused by changes in the running surface or the shoes worn by the athlete, as well as jumping and quick starts and stops.

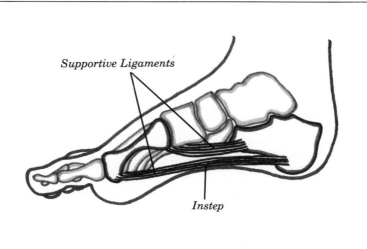

29. COMMON SITES FOR FOOT STRAIN
(Inner-side View of Foot with Supportive Ligaments)

PREVENTION:

This injury is difficult to eliminate, but properly fitting shoes can help.

TREATMENT:

The main treatment is rest, ice, and compression. An elastic support, felt pads, or taping can ease the discomfort of ordinary walking. A whirlpool bath and aspirin can also be beneficial.

RETURN TO COMPETITION:

When the young athlete can run and jump without pain. This usually takes one or two weeks.

Tendinitis

A tendon in the foot becomes swollen and painful. Foot tendinitis is an overuse injury that usually occurs in highly skilled young athletes, such as soccer players who always control the ball. It is of little concern and can be controlled with good care.

WHAT TO LOOK FOR:
Redness, swelling, pain when using foot.

CAUSE:
Tendinitis of the foot is most common in soccer, from constant kicking with the foot extended. This can cause pain and swelling in the long tendon that controls the big toe. High-jumpers, long-jumpers, sprinters, and basketball players also can develop this type of tendinitis. *Achilles* tendinitis of the heel cord is rare in young athletes.

PREVENTION:
Conditioning, training, and skill in performance can reduce these injuries but not entirely prevent them.

TREATMENT:
Tendinitis is treated with rest, ice, and taping or elastic support. With this treatment, the condition will subside in seven to ten days.

RETURN TO COMPETITION:
When tendinitis occurs, the young athlete need not interrupt competition so long as the pain is acceptable.

Foot Sprain

Foot sprain is an injury to the ligaments in the midfoot or forefoot (Illustration 30). These short, firm, thick ligaments hold together the small block-like bones that establish the arch of the foot. This acute injury discourages the best competitors, but will eventually heal without impairing athletic performance.

WHAT TO LOOK FOR:
Swelling, tenderness under the arch or over the instep, and pain when walking.

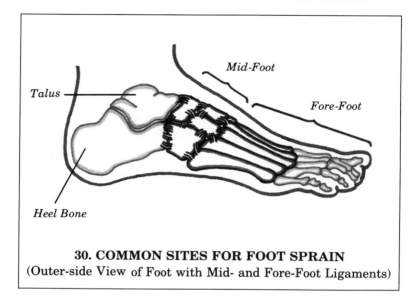

30. COMMON SITES FOR FOOT SPRAIN
(Outer-side View of Foot with Mid- and Fore-Foot Ligaments)

CAUSE:

Excessive jumping and running. The injury occurs most often to high-jumpers, and sometimes to pole-vaulters, long-jumpers, and hurdlers. It occurs more rarely in tennis and other sports.

PREVENTION:

Difficult to prevent, but conditioning and skill in performance can help.

TREATMENT:

Rest, ice, compression, crutches, and splinting of the foot when the injury is severe.

RETURN TO COMPETITION:

The torn ligaments take three to six weeks to heal (although it seems much longer to a young athlete in the middle of a season).

Do Young Athletes Need Arch Supports?

Arch supports are often recommended for young athletes to relieve pain or correct weight-bearing imbalance. In my opinion, based on examining and treating the feet of hundreds of young athletes, they rarely need arch supports. I recommend them for the adolescent foot only in exceptional cases, such as when the foot is abnormally structured, the athlete has chronic pain that doesn't respond to rest, or unusual foot and leg problems occur. If arch supports are used, it should be for only short periods, not as permanent equipment. Moreover, custom-molded arch supports are very expensive, and the youngster will most likely discard them quickly anyway.

Soccer Toe

Also known as "turf toe," this is a severe pain in the first metatarsal joint of the big toe. It's a common injury in soccer and football that is not serious but can be temporarily disabling.

WHAT TO LOOK FOR:
Swelling and pain at the base of the big toe.

CAUSE:
Pushing off with the toe while bearing the full weight of the body.

PREVENTION:
Prevention is difficult, but a properly fitted shoe can help.

TREATMENT:
Rest, ice, taping, and splinting.

There need be no interruption for mild cases, about a week for more severe cases.

Accessory Navicular Injury

This is an irritation of the accessory navicular—a small extra bone on the inner side of the mid-foot that is attached to one of the major ligaments that lift and turn the foot in such activities as kicking. This condition usually affects teenage girls. It can become a nagging problem, but eventually subsides in almost all cases.

WHAT TO LOOK FOR:
Pain and swelling in the medial area of the midfoot, and tenderness of the prominent extra bone.

CAUSE:
Running and jumping, and occasionally poorly fitted ski boots or ice skates.

PREVENTION:
No preventive measures.

TREATMENT:
This condition should be treated in the same way as tendinitis. It is one situation in which arch supports (see pg. 291) can help. Surgery should be avoided when possible. I have seen some cases in which surgery was recommended but not carried out—and after treatment, rest, and a change in the youngster's sport, there were no future problems with the condition. Surgery is a viable option when the condition is severe, but there is a risk that the operation will disrupt the balance of the foot.

RETURN TO COMPETITION:
When the pain and discomfort subside enough to permit returning.

Stress Fracture

The typical stress fracture in a youngster's foot occurs to the third metatarsal (Illustration 31), but this injury heals well with proper care. Two other stress fractures of the foot can cause complications when the injury is inadequately diagnosed or treated. One is a fracture of the navicular bone, which is located on the inside of the arch (Illustration 32). The other is a fracture at the base of the fifth metatarsal (Illustration 33). Because initial X rays do not show these fractures clearly, they are often missed and mistakenly diagnosed as sprains. If pain and disability persist without a

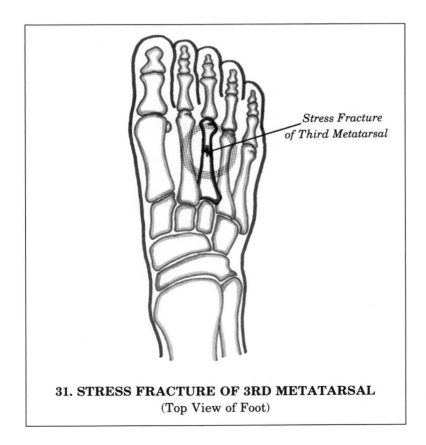

Stress Fracture of Third Metatarsal

31. STRESS FRACTURE OF 3RD METATARSAL
(Top View of Foot)

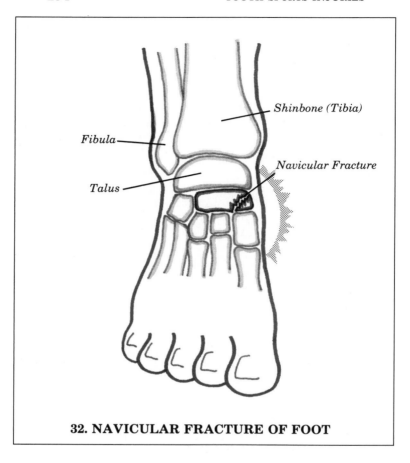

Shinbone (Tibia)

Fibula

Navicular Fracture

Talus

32. NAVICULAR FRACTURE OF FOOT

proper diagnosis, the result may be serious damage requiring major surgery.

WHAT TO LOOK FOR:
Persistent pain.

CAUSE:
This stress injury is caused by overuse, and frequently occurs in basketball.

PREVENTION:
It's difficult to prevent, but conditioning can help.

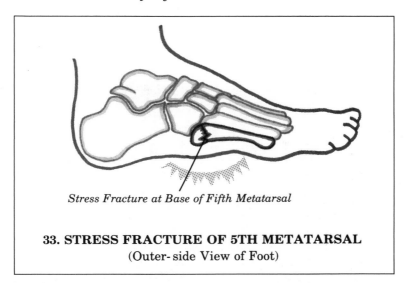

Stress Fracture at Base of Fifth Metatarsal

33. STRESS FRACTURE OF 5TH METATARSAL
(Outer- side View of Foot)

TREATMENT:
Should be treated in the same way as stress fractures of the leg (see page 279).

RETURN TO COMPETITION:
After solid healing of the bone.

Sever's Condition

This is an inflammation of the growth bone in the back of the heel (Illustration 34). It is the most common foot complaint of young male athletes between ten and thirteen years old, particularly in the spring when they start doing a lot more running than they have all winter. This is an injury of no consequence that usually goes away after a few weeks, although in rare cases the problem may persist for as long as a year.

WHAT TO LOOK FOR:
Heel pain while walking, running, or jumping, growing worse as the day goes on.

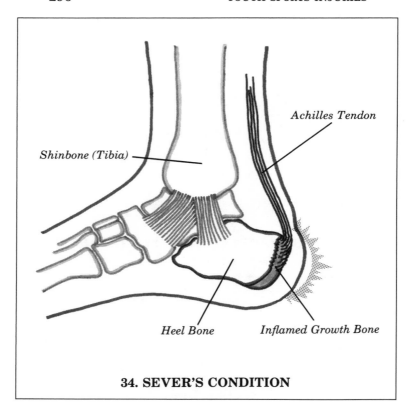

Shinbone (Tibia)

Achilles Tendon

Heel Bone

Inflamed Growth Bone

34. SEVER'S CONDITION

CAUSE:

Irritation from overuse.

PREVENTION:

No preventive measures.

TREATMENT:

Supportive treatment includes a heel pad, warm soaks, rest, and aspirin or other pain medication. If the condition is persistent, which is rare, a nonwalking cast may be necessary for three weeks. There is no need for surgery.

RETURN TO COMPETITION:
This condition usually doesn't stop a youngster from playing, even though there may be a persistent limp and complaints about the pain.

Athlete's Foot

This red, itchy inflammation between the toes is a common nuisance condition in all sports.

WHAT TO LOOK FOR:
Pain, swelling, and itching.

CAUSE:
A fungal infection.

PREVENTION:
Cleanliness, keeping feet dry, frequent change of socks, and foot powder.

TREATMENT:
Readily responds to antifungal powders and ointments.

RETURN TO COMPETITION:
No interruption in competition should be necessary.

17

Knee Injuries

◆

K nee injuries get special attention in the *Home Reference Guide* for several reasons:

- An injury to the knee is the most frequent serious extremity injury in sports.
- Knee injuries account for more time lost from competition by young athletes than any other type of injury.
- Knee injuries end more athletic careers and disable more athletes in later years than any other sports injury.
- It is sometimes difficult to determine the severity of a knee injury.
- The decisions that orthopedic surgeons make about treatment of a knee injury are critical to a young athlete's future.
- A severely injured knee is often at risk when an athlete returns to competition, even after surgery.

In short, knee injuries are the young athlete's nemesis. That's the bad news. The good news is that we are making rapid progress in understanding the secrets of the knee. Laboratory research and advances in treatment, such as arthroscopic surgery and ligament reconstruction, have expanded both our knowledge and our ability to care for knee injuries.

Because healthy knees are crucial to the success of a

young athlete and to one's fitness in later years, the *Guide* goes into considerable detail about knee injuries. This information is based on my concentration on knee injuries over more than thirty years as an orthopedic surgeon.

This section is divided into six parts:

1. Anatomy of the knee
2. Evaluating knee injuries
3. Specific knee injuries from sports
4. Knee conditions related to sports
5. Knee braces
6. Knee rehabilitation

◆ ANATOMY OF THE KNEE

As a parent of young athletes, you can profit from knowing something about the major structures that make up the knee joint. When the doctor explains an injury and discusses available treatment options, you will be better equipped to understand what is being said.

The knee looks simple from the outside, but inside it is extremely complicated. This *Guide* simplifies the knee's structure to make its important parts crystal clear.

The knee joint has a flat surface. It connects the thigh bone (*femur*) with the leg bone (*tibia*), which are not interlocked, as are the bones in the ankle or hip. The joint has these important parts (Illustrations 35 and 36):

- *Kneecap (Patella)*. This prominent disc-like bone that sits in the knee and glides over the joint is a miracle of nature. Working as a fulcrum to give the knee power for bending and straightening, it is supported by muscles and ligaments from above and by a large tendon from below.
- *Cartilage (Meniscus)*. Each knee has two *menisci*—firm, rubbery pieces of gristle shaped like a quarter-moon. The *medial meniscus* lies on the inner side of the joint, the *lateral meniscus* on the outer side. They act as shock absorbers, pro-

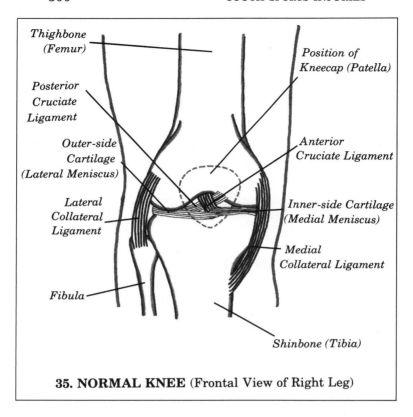

Thighbone (Femur)

Position of Kneecap (Patella)

Posterior Cruciate Ligament

Outer-side Cartilage (Lateral Meniscus)

Anterior Cruciate Ligament

Lateral Collateral Ligament

Inner-side Cartilage (Medial Meniscus)

Medial Collateral Ligament

Fibula

Shinbone (Tibia)

35. NORMAL KNEE (Frontal View of Right Leg)

viding a cushion to the knee joint. In recent years, they have also been recognized as important supporting structures.

• *Ligaments.* These are the strong, thick, fibrous structures that hold the joint and the bones together, but are not directly connected to muscles. Four major ligaments maintain the knee's stability.

1. **Anterior Cruciate Ligament (ACL).** Short and round, this is the critical supporting ligament, keeping the knee tight and providing maximum stability. To get an idea of what this ligament does, squeeze your right thumb tightly with your left hand. At the same time that the ligament prevents slippage within the joint, it permits the joint to pivot.

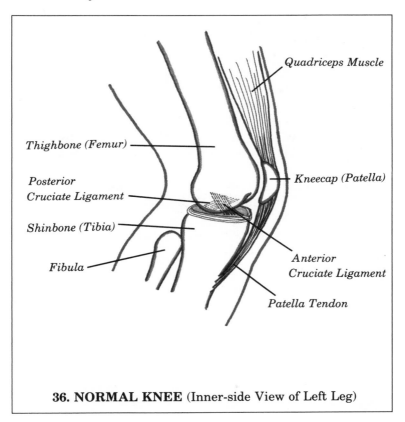

36. NORMAL KNEE (Inner-side View of Left Leg)

2. **Medial Collateral Ligament (MCL).** This is a broad, flat, powerful ligament with two layers that hold the inner side of the knee joint tight. It also supports the *medial meniscus* and protects the side of the knee.
3. **Lateral Collateral Ligament (LCL).** This ligament consists of three structures that help to stabilize the outside of the knee joint. The *lateral meniscus* is closely connected to this ligament.
4. **Posterior Cruciate Ligament (PCL).** This short, powerful ligament is located in the back of the knee joint behind the *anterior cruciate* and supports the back structures of the knee. Its function is to help stabilize the knee.

◆ EVALUATING KNEE INJURIES

Rule one in evaluating knee injuries is: *Do it as soon as possible after the injury has occurred.* It is best to examine the knee on the sidelines or in the locker room before there is pain, spasm, and swelling. A young athlete should not be allowed to continue playing with a knee injury until it is examined, in order to prevent further damage that could have been avoided by recognizing the seriousness of the injury.

Rule two is: *Have the immediate evaluation done by an expert.* This can be either a skilled trainer or a physician familiar with knee injuries.

The first step is to examine the knee and get answers to these questions:

- How much swelling is there?
- Is the swelling in the tissue outside or inside the knee joint? (This can be determined by feeling the knee.)
- Is the knee painful to touch? If so, where?
- Is there pain and apprehension when the kneecap is moved from side to side?
- Can the knee be straightened out all the way?
- Does it completely bend or is it locked?
- Is there any looseness on the inside or outside of the joint?

A more thorough evaluation of the injury should be done in a clinic or doctor's office. Because knee injuries are difficult to diagnose, the examining doctor has to be something of a detective probing for clues. Part of this process is to get a complete history of the injury by asking such questions as:

- What position were you playing?
- Was the injury caused by a hit or by twisting the knee?
- Did it happen without contact with another player?
- Did the knee come out of place?
- Did the knee*cap* jump out of place?

- When the injury occurred, did you hear a "pop," grinding, crunching, or snapping?
- How severe was the pain?
- Does it hurt anywhere else besides the knee?
- How long did it take the knee to swell—an hour or not until the next day?
- Could you walk on it right away?
- Did you keep playing after the injury?
- Just after the injury, could you bend the knee all the way, slightly, or not at all?
- Is it locked or unlocked now?

Answers to these questions will help the physician to appraise the knee injury accurately.

A careful examination should follow the history. There are simple tests for determining injuries to the medial collateral, lateral collateral, and posterior cruciate ligaments. For injuries to the anterior cruciate, which can be the most serious, the best method is the Lachman test. Although not a sophisticated test, it must be conducted by an expert. The knee is bent slightly at about fifteen degrees and the leg is rocked with one hand below the knee and one holding the thigh. If there is a tear of the anterior cruciate ligament, a slipping sensation will be felt as the knee is rocked. (Medical engineers have designed a machine that will also perform this test.)

When the knee is severely swollen or painful, it may be difficult to conduct an accurate examination because of the pain, muscle spasm, and anxiety. In these cases, the examination should be conducted while the young athlete is under anesthesia. At the same time, an arthroscopic examination should be conducted. This may seem an extreme measure, but it is essential for resolving any doubts about the extent of the injury.

◆ SPECIFIC KNEE INJURIES

Contusion

This is a bruise to the knee. Although most knee bruises are minor, they should be evaluated thoroughly to make sure there is nothing seriously wrong.

WHAT TO LOOK FOR:
Pain, swelling, tenderness, black-and-blue marks.

CAUSE:
A direct blow to the kneecap.

PREVENTION:
Kneepads.

TREATMENT:
Immediate treatment is ice, compression, and support. This should be followed by exercise of the quadriceps muscle to prevent loss of strength during healing.

RETURN TO COMPETITION:
Interruption of competition may not be necessary, but a severe bruise may require a week's layoff to allow healing.

Traumatic Bursitis (Water on the Knee)

In football and volleyball, players sometimes suffer bruises in which blood collects just under the skin of the knee but not inside the joint itself. This injury looks frightening but is of little consequence.

WHAT TO LOOK FOR:
There is moderate pain and the kneecap area is squishy.

CAUSE:
A single blow or repeated impact from landing on the knee.

PREVENTION:
Kneepads.

TREATMENT:
The best treatment is ice and compression. When the injury is severe, the fluid can be drained by a physician.

RETURN TO COMPETITION:
The young athlete may keep playing, but should wear a felt pad to protect the knee. If the condition persists, it can be corrected at the end of the season.

Knee Sprain

This injury occurs when either the medial or lateral ligament is stretched. Like other sprains, a knee sprain is not serious and will heal with proper treatment. However, apparent sprains must be carefully diagnosed, because they often turn out to be cartilage tears or serious ligament injuries. Recognizing the difference is never easy, even for medical experts. However, if it's a sprain, the knee is not excessively swollen and is always stable. Stability can be checked with the Lachman test and other examination methods. Once these tests have shown that the knee is stable, the young athlete can feel confident about competing again after the sprain has healed.

WHAT TO LOOK FOR:
Some pain about the knee on the inside.

CAUSE:
A forceful twisting or wrenching (sometimes caused by a blow).

PREVENTION:

Difficult to prevent but strength training of the legs can minimize the possibility.

TREATMENT:

The young athlete should immediately stop playing and be treated with ice, compression, support, and elevation until an accurate evaluation has been made.

RETURN TO COMPETITION:

If the injury is mild, competition can resume after a few days' rest, so long as the trainer tapes and supports the knee. But if there's any question about the severity of the injury, a thorough evaluation must be made before the player can return to action.

Cartilage (Meniscus) Injury

The cartilage tears after being pinched or squeezed in the joint between the two leg bones (Illustration 37). This injury is the classic "trick knee" that has plagued so many athletes through the years. However, improved treatment has reduced its disabling potential for young athletes.

WHAT TO LOOK FOR:

The knee gives way, snaps, and sometimes locks. The locking occurs when the cartilage is caught between the knee bones and jams the joint so the knee cannot bend or straighten out. When there is only partial locking, the knee may spontaneously lock and unlock. Even a slight tear can cause difficulty and give the athlete a feeling of insecurity when running, cutting, turning, or stopping suddenly.

CAUSE:

The knee is wrenched or twisted on itself.

PREVENTION:

None.

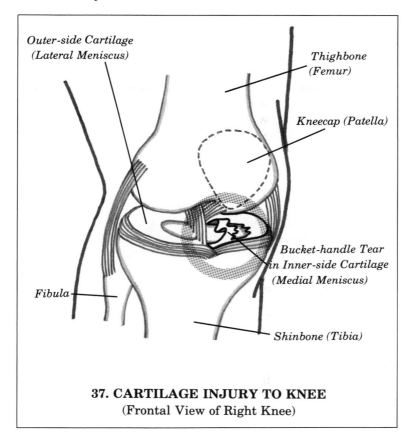

Outer-side Cartilage
(Lateral Meniscus)

Thighbone
(Femur)

Kneecap (Patella)

Bucket-handle Tear
in Inner-side Cartilage
(Medial Meniscus)

Fibula

Shinbone (Tibia)

37. CARTILAGE INJURY TO KNEE
(Frontal View of Right Knee)

TREATMENT:

The first step is to determine that there are no torn ligaments or other injuries to the knee. This is done by careful history, physical examination, an X ray, and in some cases, an MRI or arthrogram. The MRI is non-invasive and there is no radiation exposure.

Treatment of a torn cartilage has changed radically since 1975 with the development of arthroscopic surgery. Previously, the entire cartilage was surgically removed, frequently resulting in early degenerative arthritis. Now a surgeon can examine the damage inside the knee joint with a pencil-sized telescope, called an arthroscope, inserted through a small incision in the joint. Using this arthroscope, the surgeon can then insert instruments and operate on the knee, either removing just the damaged fragment or repairing the torn cartilage with sutures. With this technique, there is minimal damage to the joint and the prognosis is good for a young athlete to continue competing. This method provides the best possible care for a torn cartilage.

RETURN TO COMPETITION:

In some cases, a young athlete may be able to continue competing with no disability or loss of skill from the torn cartilage. But in most cases, any attempt to continue will put the knee in greater jeopardy. If the young athlete does get permission to keep playing, the knee should be taped and, in some cases, protected by a brace.

When the young athlete discontinues play and undergoes arthroscopic surgery to repair the torn cartilage, competition may be resumed as soon as three weeks. The exact timing must be left up to the surgeon.

Anterior Cruciate Ligament (ACL) Injury

The anterior cruciate ligament is torn (Illustrations 38 and 39). This ligament is the key to a healthy knee, and when it is injured, the knee is never the same. The injury does not seem to be related to size, strength, or weight—both the smallest female field hockey player and the massive football lineman tear this ligament.

WHAT TO LOOK FOR:

A "pop," pain, sometimes rapid swelling, a feeling the knee "came apart."

CAUSE:

The injury usually occurs when:

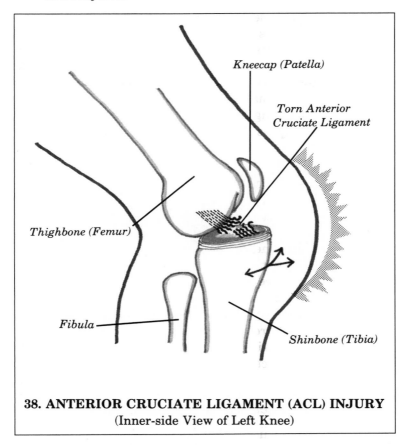

38. ANTERIOR CRUCIATE LIGAMENT (ACL) INJURY
(Inner-side View of Left Knee)

- The athlete is running, plants a leg, and quickly pivots.
- The knee receives a blow, wrenching open the joint.
- The athlete lands after a broad jump, basketball jump, or hitting a bump in a ski run.

PREVENTION:

Not really preventable, but strength training can help.

TREATMENT:

When an anterior cruciate tear is diagnosed, you and your athlete must decide whether to go ahead with

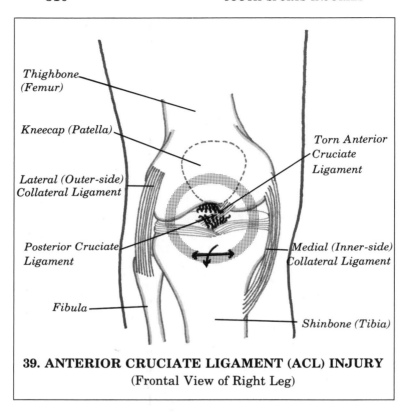

Thighbone
(Femur)

Kneecap (Patella)

Lateral (Outer-side)
Collateral Ligament

Posterior Cruciate
Ligament

Fibula

Torn Anterior
Cruciate
Ligament

Medial (Inner-side)
Collateral Ligament

Shinbone (Tibia)

39. ANTERIOR CRUCIATE LIGAMENT (ACL) INJURY
(Frontal View of Right Leg)

surgery. First, make sure your child's knee injury is in
the hands of an orthopedic surgeon who specializes in
knee-ligament repairs. Find a surgeon with solid experience and a good reputation who is willing to refer
you to the families of young athletes whose knee injuries he or she has successfully repaired. Don't hesitate to ask how many knee operations the surgeon has
performed in the past year.

Get a complete explanation of the treatment
choices—and a second opinion from another knee surgeon if you think it's needed. Be sure to involve your
youngster in these discussions and in the decisions that
are to be made. If you press your child for surgery and

the results are not what the youngster expected, you may be in for a great deal of resentment.

Several surgical techniques are used for reconstructing knee ligaments. Most knee surgeons will have expertise in one of these methods, which they use because they get good results. Today, the success rate for ACL reconstructions is around 85 to 90 percent— a major improvement over the rate of just a few years ago. But keep in mind that, as with any surgical procedure, the variables are great: genes, elasticity of body tissue, unforeseen difficulties. Moreover, despite advances, medical science has not yet mastered the anatomy of the knee.

What about the timing of ACL surgery? Most knee surgeons, including myself, believe that the knee should be given a chance to recover from the initial injury, so that it can regain normal motion and strength before surgery is performed. However, there are differences of opinion among knee specialists.

A successful ACL operation can stabilize the knee sufficiently for a youngster to continue in competitive sports. However, you and your young athlete may decide to defer surgery or not have it at all. In that case, the knee will remain unstable and probably suffer more damage. Even if your youngster gives up sports, the knee may continue to come apart just from daily activity.

On the other hand, there are some youngsters who don't have surgery and can still participate in sports.

RETURN TO COMPETITION:
Return is indicated when the knee is strong and stable, and the young athlete can run and cut without problems—which takes between nine and twelve months after surgery.

Medial Collateral Ligament (MCL) Injury

The MCL is the most vulnerable ligament. It can be torn from one of three points: the upper thigh bone (*femur*), the center at the joint, or the leg bone (Illustration 40). However, isolated medial collateral injuries heal well with no residual weakness or instability.

WHAT TO LOOK FOR:

The knee is loose and painful to the touch on the inner side.

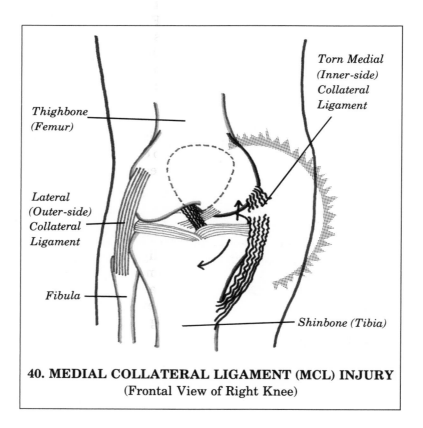

40. MEDIAL COLLATERAL LIGAMENT (MCL) INJURY
(Frontal View of Right Knee)

CAUSE:

The medial collateral is stretched when the athlete plants a foot and changes direction. This usually results in a sprain, but when there is excessive twisting force, the stretch can become a tear. This injury can also be caused by a blow to the knee.

PREVENTION:

Some high schools are using protective braces to prevent this injury, but so far their value is unproven.

TREATMENT:

MCL tears should be treated with rest, ice, compression, and, in some cases, a splint. Follow-up care should include whirlpool baths, exercises, and protection with a brace that permits limited motion of the knee joint. This injury seldom requires surgery, unless other ligaments are damaged at the same time.

RETURN TO COMPETITION:

Caution should be used, and each injury should be considered individually. Returning to competition too soon can result in a more extensive tear. Only a qualified physician should decide.

Lateral Collateral Ligament (LCL) Injury

In a tear of the lateral collateral ligament the nerve to the foot may also be stretched and damaged. This injury is not nearly so frequent as medial and anterior ligament injuries, which is fortunate, because a severe tear can result in permanent nerve damage, causing a partial paralysis called "drop foot."

WHAT TO LOOK FOR:

Pain, swelling, and instability (causing the knee to slip in and out of place).

CAUSE:

Usually caused by a violent twist, a blow from a football block, or another player accidentally falling on the knee while it is twisted into an awkward position.

PREVENTION:

Difficult to prevent.

TREATMENT:

Lateral ligament tears almost always require surgical reconstruction.

RETURN TO COMPETITION:

Only after a solid recovery, when the leg has regained strength and the young athlete can run and cut without difficulty.

Posterior Cruciate Ligament (PCL) Injury

A tear of the posterior cruciate, located in the back of the knee joint, is an uncommon injury that usually occurs without the involvement of other ligaments. It happens primarily in football, basketball, and skiing and can be disabling.

WHAT TO LOOK FOR:

Unusual looseness and a feeling that something is wrong—but these symptoms may not show up right away, making the injury difficult to diagnose immediately.

CAUSE:

A blow or certain kinds of twisting.

PREVENTION:

None.

TREATMENT:

There are two schools of thought on the preferred treatment of PCL tears. I belong to the school that believes this tear needs surgical repair only if other ligaments are involved. Other orthopedic surgeons believe that all PCL tears should be repaired.

If the initial diagnosis is missed, delayed reconstruction is inadvisable unless the injury is seriously disabling, because it is a complicated operation that does not always give satisfactory results. It is possible for athletes with this injury to be active in sports, usually with the support of a knee brace.

RETURN TO COMPETITION:
When the knee is stable and the athlete can run and cut.

Dislocated Knee Joint

The entire knee joint is completely displaced. This disastrous injury is thankfully rare—I see an average of one dislocation every seven years. When it does occur, an amputation at the knee may be necessary if the proper care is not given immediately. Knee dislocations usually occur in football and basketball, but are possible in any contact/collision sport.

WHAT TO LOOK FOR:
Excruciating pain, deformity, and loss of circulation to the leg.

CAUSE:
A major blow to the leg or a sudden, forceful twist.

PREVENTION:
No preventive measures.

TREATMENT:
This is a red-flag emergency requiring immediate intervention by a surgical team that includes an orthopedic surgeon and a vascular surgeon. Any delay can be catastrophic.

RETURN TO COMPETITION:

Return to any serious sports competition is unlikely after this serious injury.

Acute Kneecap Dislocation

The kneecap comes out of its groove, ending up on the side of the knee joint (Illustration 41). Even when treated properly, this acute injury can cause chronic instability of the kneecap (see next page). It is most common in basketball, but can occur in any sport.

WHAT TO LOOK FOR:

Severe pain, swelling, and deformity.

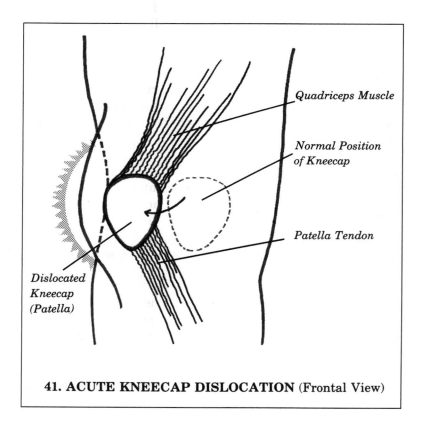

Quadriceps Muscle

Normal Position of Kneecap

Patella Tendon

Dislocated Kneecap (Patella)

41. ACUTE KNEECAP DISLOCATION (Frontal View)

CAUSE:

Direct blows and quick pivots or twists.

PREVENTION:

Not really preventable, but strength training of the quadriceps muscle may help.

TREATMENT:

Immediate care should include ice, compression, and a splint. Sometimes the kneecap goes back in place on its own, but in other cases it must be put back by an orthopedic surgeon. Most surgeons will put the kneecap in a cast or brace for several weeks, after which physical therapy is administered. Others recommend immediate surgical repair. I opt for the first, more conservative method, which usually brings satisfactory results.

RETURN TO COMPETITION:

When the quadriceps muscle is strong and the kneecap appears stable. The young athlete should wear a brace while competing.

Unstable Kneecap (Patella)

Loose ligaments cause the kneecap to slip off the outside edge of the joint during sports activity. This chronic condition—also called a subluxing or dislocating kneecap—is caused by physical abnormalities or an acute injury. It takes much time and care to correct.

WHAT TO LOOK FOR:

The knee buckles in pain, and there is a sensation of something going out of place. Sometimes the young athlete can actually see the kneecap going in and out.

CAUSE:

A blow, twist, or any one of several abnormalities, including:

- The groove in the knee joint may be too shallow.
- The outside of the groove is underdeveloped.
- The young athlete may be "knocked-kneed," causing the kneecap to pull sideways rather than up and down.
- Weak muscles and ligaments on one side of the kneecap.
- The kneecap may be too small.
- The kneecap may be located too high or too low within the joint.

These are known reasons for kneecap instability—in some cases there may not be any apparent cause.

PREVENTION:
No preventive measures.

TREATMENT:
To diagnose this condition, most doctors use a simple, foolproof method called the apprehension test. The doctor holds the kneecap gently and begins to move it to one side suddenly. When the young athlete feels that the kneecap is going to slip out of place and grabs the doctor's hand, the doctor knows exactly what's wrong.

Once the condition is identified, exercises and bracing can help in many cases, but other cases may require surgery. The most widely used approach is arthroscopic, "lateral ligament release" surgery, which is quite successful. Open surgery is not used much today but may be necessary in difficult cases.

RETURN TO COMPETITION:
When the quadriceps muscle is strong and the kneecap appears stable. The young athlete should wear a brace while competing.

◆   KNEE CONDITIONS

My sports medical center is constantly full of aching knees. In fact, "My knee hurts," is probably the most frequent complaint I hear from young athletes. For the most part, these aches and pains are simply caused by excessive exercise and activity. This section explains a few of the more common problems.

Kneecap Strain

A complaint of pain at the kneecap and lower front area of the knee, this is one of the more mysterious sports ailments, because it is extremely difficult to discover what's wrong.

WHAT TO LOOK FOR:

Pain during certain activities, particularly squatting, jumping, and running, but occasionally others such as climbing stairs.

CAUSE:

The injury is usually caused by overuse or a subtle abnormality of the knee, such as kneecap misalignment, muscle weakness, or inflammation of the tendons and ligaments.

PREVENTION:

A conditioning program with continuous exercises of the lower extremities should help, but is not always successful in preventing this condition.

TREATMENT:

Strengthening the quadriceps muscle and avoiding the sports that trouble the knee. The youngster's knee should be checked periodically by a physician, because there could be a condition—such as *osteochondritis dissecans* (see page 327)—that is not easy to identify in the early stages. X rays could show changes over time. Periodic evaluations could also reveal whether emotional stress is responsible. (See Teen-Age Knee below)

RETURN TO COMPETITION:

When the pain has subsided.

"Teen-Age Knee" (T.A.K.)

There is nothing physically wrong. The knee is normal, without swelling, tenderness, or apparent mechanical difficulty. This is a specific type of painful knee most frequently found in girls of thirteen and fourteen, but occasionally in boys as well.

WHAT TO LOOK FOR:

Pain in the knee, usually during sports activity.

CAUSE:

Although the symptoms may be similar to those of kneecap strain, the cause of T.A.K. seems to be emotional rather than physical. A careful history may uncover pressure from family problems, peers, or the youngster's coach.

TREATMENT:

Possible alternatives are to discontinue competition for a while, change sports, or drop sports altogether. A youngster with this condition will often express relief when told "No sports for now." In some cases, professional counseling may be necessary.

RETURN TO COMPETITION:

Only when the knee pain is gone and the youngster seems to have adjusted satisfactorily. Obviously, if the knee pain returns after resumption of sports, the activity should be discontinued again.

Chondromalacia

True *chondromalacia* consists of long-standing, permanent damage to the undersurface of the kneecap, and it can cause significant disability for a young athlete. Unfortunately, this term is used much too often by those treating young athletes with knee pain, simply because there is a grinding, squeaky, or crunching noise present when the knee is moved. Noisy knees are common in youngsters, and in many cases the noise and the pain will disappear after time. The diagnosis of *chondromalacia* should be used only after accurate evaluation is carried out, including an MRI and/or arthroscopic examination.

WHAT TO LOOK FOR:

Chronic pain in or around the kneecap, associated with a grinding sensation and sometimes noise. The condition is particularly troublesome when the youngster is squatting or climbing stairs.

CAUSE:

Overuse, a blow, or a structural defect that causes the kneecap to be squeezed excessively against the knee joint.

PREVENTION:

To avoid developing this condition from overuse, the young athlete should strengthen the quadriceps muscle.

TREATMENT:

Once there is a valid diagnosis, treatment includes maintaining strength in the quadriceps and hamstrings, discontinuing sports that may aggravate the condition, applying ice when the pain is troublesome, wearing a kneecap brace, and, rarely, undergoing arthroscopic surgery to remove excess tissue. In extreme cases, more complicated surgery may be necessary. But generally with this condition, the less that is done the better.

RETURN TO COMPETITION:

Usually when completely free of complaints, but in certain cases the youngster can play if the discomfort is tolerable and not aggravated by the activity.

Osgood-Schlatter's Condition

This is an inflammation of the growth center just below the knee, where the kneecap tendon connects to the bone.

X rays may reveal characteristic bone fragmentation (Illustration 42). The active, painful inflammation can heal in six months or last for three years—in rare cases, even longer. This condition—named after the two doctors who discovered it separately and simultaneously in 1903—is of little consequence. Even though it may persist for a few years, it almost always heals. It's usually a complaint of boys between eleven and fourteen, and occasionally of girls. Having "oscars," as these youngsters call it, seems to be a painful but popular status symbol on young teams.

WHAT TO LOOK FOR:

Pain, growing more intense when the knee is hit or overused.

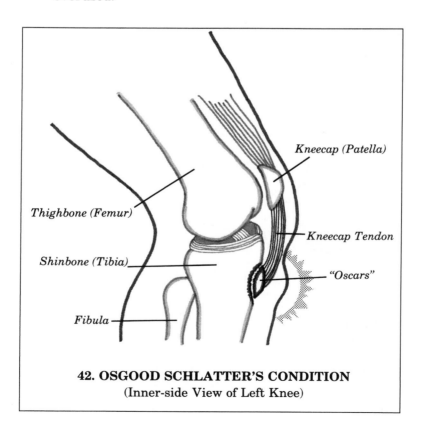

42. OSGOOD SCHLATTER'S CONDITION
(Inner-side View of Left Knee)

CAUSE:

Overuse.

PREVENTION:

None.

TREATMENT:

Rest, ice, and aspirin are best. Taping a felt "doughnut" pad around the swelling can be helpful in collision sports. Avoid a cast, which can weaken the thigh muscles and endanger the knee. I don't recommend surgery except in rare cases when the condition persists for many years into the young athlete's twenties.

Once the condition heals, the only residual is a minor bump just below the knee. This can be permanent, but it doesn't seem to disturb most people.

RETURN TO COMPETITION:

If the condition doesn't bother your youngster, he or she can play any sport. Even if the condition causes pain or limping, it won't do any harm to continue playing if the youngster so desires.

Jumper's Knee

An inflammation of the tendon that connects the kneecap to the leg (Illustration 43), this is an overuse condition typically found among basketball players. Basketball is a sport that is played all year around, seven days a week, in school yards, on the street, at the playground, in the back yard. The game's popularity has produced many fine players, but it has also produced "jumper's knee."

A growing incidence of this condition in other sports besides basketball is very troublesome, because it is hard to eliminate. I have even seen it in ten-year-olds. One was a girl active in gymnastics, soccer, and ice skating—all in the same season. Her parents followed my advice and pulled her from sports until the condition healed, then permitted her to go back to only one of the sports.

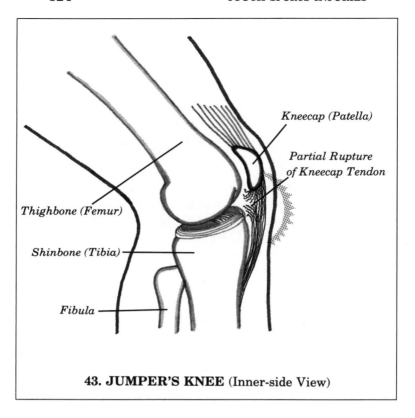

43. JUMPER'S KNEE (Inner-side View)

However, although this is a nagging condition, it is neither serious nor permanent.

WHAT TO LOOK FOR:

Pain and tenderness at the lowest point of the kneecap.

CAUSE:

Overuse in jumping.

PREVENTION:

The only prevention is to reduce sports activity.

TREATMENT:

During the off-season, the condition should be treated with rest (no running or jumping), ice massage, and exercise of the quadriceps and lower leg. Be warned that this will not sit well with your youngster, because it may take many weeks of this treatment before the pain subsides.

During the season, the choice is to play with the pain or stop playing and treat the pain with rest and ice. Anti-inflammatories should be limited to over-the-counter medicines such as acetaminophen or aspirin. I don't prescribe any anti-inflammatory medications for these youngsters because of the danger of side effects. The most important point is, your youngster may compete with jumper's knee with no fear of further damage.

Surgical excision of the injured part of the kneecap tendon is usually quite successful, but it's rarely necessary for high-school athletes.

RETURN TO COMPETITION:
If the pain is tolerable, the young athlete may continue to play.

Split Kneecap (Bipartite Patella)

When the kneecap develops, the portion of bone in its upper outer corner fails to join the main bone (Illustration 44). When X-rayed, the kneecap appears to be in two pieces. In most cases, this extra bone causes no problem. But in some cases, the bone moves against the main kneecap, causing friction and pain.

This problem is uncommon in sports and occurs mostly in hurdles and the high jump. It is not usually serious, but sometimes requires surgery.

WHAT TO LOOK FOR:
Pain when jumping, squatting, and sometimes running.

CAUSE:
It's a congenital defect, but can be aggravated by overuse.

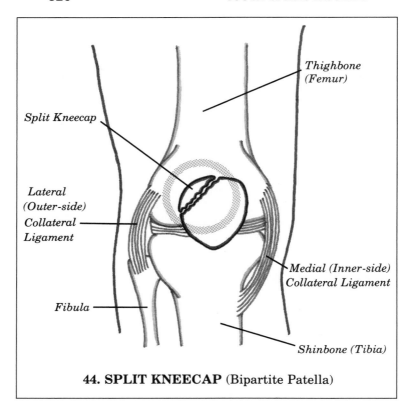

44. SPLIT KNEECAP (Bipartite Patella)

PREVENTION:
None—you're born with it.

TREATMENT:
Ice, exercise, and a kneecap strap or brace. In severe, painful cases, the only solution is to remove the fragment surgically.

RETURN TO COMPETITION:
If pain permits, competition can continue. After surgery, a young athlete can return when rehabilitation is complete.

Osteochondritis Dissecans

A fragment of bone within the joint becomes isolated and loses its blood supply (Illustration 45). In severe cases, the fragment breaks away from the joint and floats loose inside the knee. This can be a serious condition causing prolonged interruption of sports activity.

WHAT TO LOOK FOR:

Knee pain, possibly with clicking and snapping sounds. When the bone fragment has broken completely loose, there may be swelling, locking, and buckling, similar to the symptoms of a torn cartilage. At times the athlete

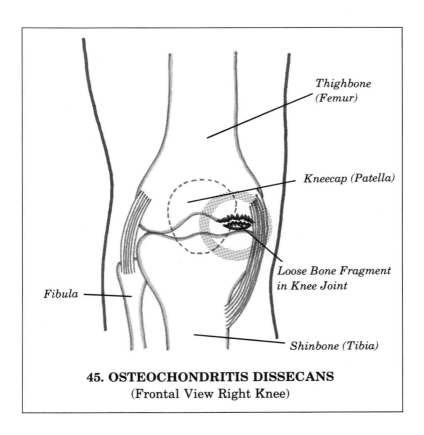

Thighbone (Femur)

Kneecap (Patella)

Loose Bone Fragment in Knee Joint

Fibula

Shinbone (Tibia)

45. OSTEOCHONDRITIS DISSECANS
(Frontal View Right Knee)

or the doctor may be able to feel the bone fragment moving around in the joint.

CAUSE:

There is no clear cause, but orthopedic surgeons generally agree that it is an overuse injury.

PREVENTION:

Difficult to prevent, because this injury is unpredictable.

TREATMENT:

Initial treatment is to restrict activity until an X ray shows that it has healed. The healing process can take months, sometimes a whole year.

Recently, an arthroscopic surgical procedure has become successful in which the fragment is held in place with small pins until healing occurs. On some occasions, the fragment may be pinned back in place even when floating loose. However, in other cases, if the fragment has been floating loose for some time, it must be removed with arthroscopic surgery.

RETURN TO COMPETITION:

When X rays show healing of the condition or after surgical removal of the fragment and physical rehabilitation.

Knee Pain Due to Hip Condition

A young athlete may have a vague, sometimes disabling knee pain that is actually caused by a major condition of the hip, such as *synovitis, Legg-Perthes disease, slipped capital ephiphysis*, a stress fracture, or a tumor. Any youngsters with knee pain that cannot be traced to a knee condition or injury should have their hips carefully examined and X-rayed. Vague pain on the outside of the knee may also be sciatic pain from a lumbar disc problem.

◆ KNEE BRACES

Protective knee braces come in two basic varieties: those used to protect knees that have been injured and those used to protect normal knees.

Braces for Injured Knees

Most knees that have been injured should be protected from further injury by some kind of brace, especially in sports that involve pivoting, turning, and sudden starting and stopping. Here's a rundown on the five basic types of knee braces that can be used:

1. *Elastic Support.* A pullover or wrap-around brace with no side hinges or rigid support. This is a minimal brace that can be used for mildly sprained knees that are still stable.
2. *Elastic Strap Support.* This wrap-around Velcro brace is stronger than a simple elastic brace but does not protect unstable knees.
3. *Kneecap Brace.* This brace uses Velcro straps to stabilize unstable kneecaps.
4. *Hinge Brace.* This widely used brace supports the knee with metal or fiberglass hinges on both sides of the knee. Excellent for sprains with medial or lateral ligament injuries.
5. *Functional Brace.* This multiple-hinged brace has front and back supports to protect the unstable knee by limiting excess pivoting and rotation during running and cutting. This is the brace of choice for protecting surgically repaired knees, particularly when the anterior cruciate ligament has been involved.

You may have to keep after your youngster to wear a knee brace when it is needed—many young athletes stop wearing them because of the inconvenience. Although there's no guarantee that knee braces can protect an unstable knee, they can significantly reduce the chances of reinjury.

Braces for Normal Knees

Researchers have developed several braces to protect normal knees in football and other collision/contact sports. These braces have a single hinge on the outer side of the knee. To be of any benefit, they must be custom-tailored to the individual athlete and properly fitted with each wearing.

As of this writing, the value of braces for the normal knee has not been proven. Although some clinical research indicates that they will prevent or reduce knee injuries, the American Association of Orthopedic Surgeons has called the research unsound. Moreover, some studies suggest that other types of injuries, such as ankle sprains, may *increase* with the use of these braces.

◆ KNEE REHABILITATION

More than with any other joint, it is absolutely critical for the knee joint to be completely rehabilitated before a youngster returns to competition. This means not only healing, but recovering normal strength, agility, and confidence. When a knee is splinted and unexercised, the quadriceps muscle can lose one inch in two weeks.

Here are some basic guidelines for knee rehabilitation programs:

1. They should be planned and supervised by a certified trainer or registered physical therapist working together with a physician.
2. To prevent atrophy, a rehab program should start the next day after an injury or after surgery.
3. Before competition can resume, the injured knee must have recovered at least 85 percent of its power compared with the other knee.
4. The young athlete must have a full range of motion before returning to competition. This includes being able to sprint, do agility exercises, squat comfortably, and extend the leg straight without wobbling.

A

Medical Terms: A Glossary

◆

accessory navicular: a secondary bone adjacent to the navicular bone of the foot.

achilles tendon: the large tendon, called the heel cord, at the heel of the foot.

acromion: bony prominence that projects over the shoulder and connects with the collarbone at the acromio-clavicular joint.

acute injury: a sudden injury, such as one caused by a blow.

amenorrhea: absence of menstrual periods.

anabolic steroids: synthetic forms of the male hormone testosterone; used to promote muscle mass.

angulation of a fracture: the bending at an angle of a broken bone.

anorexia nervosa: a refusal to eat, often caused by a psychological problem.

anterior: toward the front; e.g., the anterior cruciate ligament is at the front of the knee.

anterior compartment syndrome: massive swelling of the anterior muscle compartment of the leg.

anterior cruciate ligament: a major ligament located in the central anterior region of the knee.

arthrogram: an examination technique in which dye is injected into a joint, which is then X-rayed.

arthroscopy: another examination technique, in which a small telescope, attached to a television camera, is inserted into the joint.

asthma: a disorder causing difficulty in breathing.

atrophy: wasting away of a muscle or other part of the body.

avulsion fracture: a fracture in which part of a bone is forcefully torn away.

Bankart operation: a surgical procedure that stabilizes the shoulder joint. Named after the British surgeon who first used the procedure in 1923.

bone scan: a test in which radioactive material is injected into the body. The test shows increased radioactivity in the area of an abnormal bone condition such as a stress fracture.

Bristow procedure: a surgical procedure that uses a bone block to reconstruct a dislocating shoulder.

bulimia: an eating disorder characterized by gobbling large quantities of food and then vomiting.

bursitis: inflammation of the *bursa*, a soft, fluid-filled sac that minimizes friction near joints, such as the shoulder and knee joints.

cartilage: the surface tissue of any joint, but particularly the meniscus of the knee joint.

CAT scan: a computerized X-ray technique that provides extraordinary pictures of parts of the body in thin slices.

chondromalacia: a softening of cartilage.

clavicle: the bone that connects the chest to the shoulder, commonly known as the collarbone.

concussion: a head injury involving brain impairment, such as disturbed vision and altered consciousness.

contusion: a bruise.

coracoid-clavicular ligament: the ligament connecting the coracoid process to the clavicle at the shoulder.

costo-chondral joints: numerous small joints that connect the ribs to the chest plate (sternum).

CPR: cardiopulmonary resuscitation, an emergency maneuver used to restore breathing and the heartbeat.

cuboid: a small bone in the mid-foot.

cuneiform: a small bone in the mid-foot.

cystic fibrosis: a hereditary disease affecting the lungs and other organs.

deltoid ligament: the ligament on the inner side of the ankle.

dislocation: displacement of the bones of a joint.

Ehlers-Danlos syndrome: a congenital condition involving excessive fragility and laxity of the skin and joints.

electromyograph (EMG): an instrument for recording electrical currents associated with muscular activity.

EMT (Emergency Medical Technician): a technician trained and qualified to respond to medical emergencies.

epiphysis: the growth center of a bone.

epicondyles: the bony prominences on the inner and outer sides of the elbow.

epidural hematoma: a collection of blood between the *dura* lining of the brain and the skull bone.

epilepsy: a disorder characterized by convulsions due to brain dysfunction.

femur: the large thigh bone connecting the hip and knee joints.

fibula: the smaller of the two leg bones.

fracture: a break in a bone.

fungus infection: an infection caused by a microorganism that affects the skin.

growth plates: centers of growth in the long bones of the body near the joints.

hamstring: massive muscle in the back of the thigh.

heart murmur: an abnormal sound given off by the heart.

hemarthrosis: a collection of blood in a joint.

hematoma: a collection of blood in the body, due to abnormal bleeding.

hemorrhage: heavy or uncontrollable bleeding.

herniation of the intervertebral disc: protuberance of tissue between the back vertebrae, frequently pressing on the sciatic nerve.

humerus: the large bone that connects the shoulder to the elbow.

hypermobility: abnormal looseness of a joint.

hypertension: abnormally high blood pressure.

hypertrophic cardiomyopathy: a congenital condition of the heart muscles.

hypothermia: loss of body temperature from exposure to cold.

ibuprofen: an anti-inflammatory medicine.

iliac crest: the high bony prominence of the iliac bone that can be felt above the hip joint.

infectious mononucleosis: a virus infection.

kyphosis: a humpback.

Lachman test: a test to determine if the anterior cruciate ligament of the knee has been damaged.

lateral: on the outer side of the body; e.g., *lateral* ligament.

lateral collateral ligament: the ligament on the outer side of the knee joint.

lateral malleolus: the outside bone of the ankle.

lateral meniscus: the cartilage located between the bones on the outer side of the knee joint, acting like a shock absorber.

Legg-Perthes: a hip disease in children characterized by loss of circulation in the head of the femur and deformity of the joint.

ligament: fibrous tissue that holds a joint together.

lordosis: abnormal curvature of the spine; swayback.

lumbar vertebrae: bones in the lower back.

medial: on the inner side of the body; e.g., *medial* ligament.

medial meniscus: the cartilage on the inner side of the knee.

metacarpal: a bone in the hand that connects to a finger bone.

metacarpal-phalangeal joint: the joint between the hand and the finger, also called the knuckle joint.

metatarsus: the fore-foot area where the metatarsal bones are located.

MRI: Magnetic Resonance Imaging—a radiological test that shows damaged and abnormal tissue in the body.

Myelogram: an X-ray study of the spinal canal taken after dye has been placed in the canal.

myositis ossificans: bony formation of muscle.

navicular: a bone located in the wrist and also in the foot.

olecranon: the prominent bone at the back of the elbow.

ophthalmologist: a physician specializing in eye examination and surgery.

oral surgeon: a dentist specializing in surgery of the teeth and mouth.

orbit: the bony socket of the eye.

orthotics: the use of mechanical supports for weak or ineffective joints or muscles.

Osgood-Schlatter's condition: inflammation of the growth center where the kneecap tendon connects to the tibia.

osteoarthritis: arthritis marked by degeneration of the joints.

osteochondritis dissecans: damage to cartilage and adjacent bone within a joint, causing loss of circulation to the bone. In some cases, a fragment of bone may become free in the joint.

osteogenesis imperfecta: a congenital disease of bone and connective tissue, resulting in very fragile bones.

paraplegia: paralysis of the muscles and nerves from the waist down.

patella: the kneecap.

pediatrician: a physician specializing in care of children.

phalanges: bones of the fingers and toes.

plastic surgeon: a specialist in cosmetic surgery.

podiatrist: a specialist in foot problems.

posterior: in back of the body.

proximal inter-phalangeal joint: the finger joint closest to the hand, between the first and second bones.

quadriceps: the massive muscle in the front part of the thigh.

quadriplegia: paralysis from the neck down.

radius: one of the two bones in the forearm that connect the elbow to the wrist.

RDA: recommended daily allowance of a nutrient.

rehabilitation: the process of helping an injured athlete recover strength and agility.

rotator cuff: the large, flat shoulder tendon that facilitates circular motion of the shoulder.

scaphoid: a bone in the wrist or foot; also called a *navicular*.

Scheuermann's disease: an inflammatory condition of the

growth centers of the spine, usually in the thoracic area, but sometimes in the lumbar area.

sciatic nerve: the large nerve going from the spinal cord all the way down to the foot.

scoliosis: a lateral curvature of the spine.

seizure: a convulsion with uncontrollable jerking of the arms and legs, caused by an imbalance in the nervous system.

separation: coming apart of a joint; e.g., shoulder separation.

Sever's condition: an inflammation of the heel bone.

slipped capital femoral epiphysis: displacement of the head of the thighbone (femur) at the hip joint before growth is complete.

spinal cord: the central mass of nerves located within the spinal canal of the vertebrae.

spleen: organ in the abdomen that forms blood cells.

spondylolisthesis: a fracture or congenital defect in the struts of the backbone.

sternoclavicular joint: the joint that connects the collarbone and the chest plate.

subdural hematoma: collection of blood under the lining of the brain, just over the brain itself.

subluxation: a partial dislocation or slipping in and out of the bone of a joint, most commonly in the shoulder.

subungual hematoma: a collection of blood under a fingernail or toenail.

synovitis: inflammation of a joint.

talus: the bone connecting the ankle to the foot; the "keystone" bone.

tendinitis: inflammation of a tendon.

tibia: the large leg bone between the knee and ankle.

traction: a pulling or stretching.

transverse process: the lateral strut projecting from the vertebrae; the backbone.

ulna: one of the two bones in the forearm connecting the elbow to the wrist.

vertebrae: the bony or cartilaginous segments composing the spinal column.

B

Locker Room Jargon: A Glossary

◆

Young athletes have a language all their own. When your youngster comes home and tells you "I was clotheslined," or "I have a horse kiss," all you may be able to respond is "Huh?" The following glossary will help you to decipher these and other unfamiliar phrases you're likely to hear.

baseball finger: a rupture of the tendon of the last joint of the finger, resulting in a dropped appearance of the fingertip.

bell ringer: a blow to the head that may have caused a concussion. Also heard as "My bell was rung."

biker's knee: pain in and around the kneecap caused by excessive stress in long-distance cycling.

biker's palsy: numbness and tingling in the fourth and fifth fingers, caused by gripping the handlebars for long periods.

black toe: a condition of distance runners in which the nail bed of one or more toes turns black from repeated injury.

blocker's arm: hard swelling in the arm from constant hitting while blocking in football.

boxer's fracture: a depressed knuckle fracture caused by a punch.

breast-stroke knee: pain that develops on the inner side of the knee from doing the breast stroke in swimming.

buddy taping: treating an injured finger by taping it to the adjacent finger.

burner: tingling, numbness, and pain from the shoulder to the hand, caused in football by an injury to the neck or upper shoulder.

butt blocking: See *spearing.*

cauliflower ear: a swelling on the upper edge or in the lobe of the ear, caused in wrestling when the ear is crushed or rubbed on the mat.

clotheslining: stiff-arming a ball-carrier in football to throw him off his feet. A dangerous maneuver that is now outlawed.

dead arm: an arm that is disabled for a few seconds to a few minutes because of an unstable shoulder that subluxes or dislocates.

ding: see *bell ringer.*

face blocking: using one's face mask to hit an opposing player in football.

frog: a muscle spasm or cramp caused by a direct blow.

glass arm: see *dead arm.*

goring: see *spearing.*

hammer toe: a toe that is curled up in a fixed position with a callus on top of the knuckle.

handlebar palsy: see *biker's palsy.*

helmet bump: a bump in the center of one's forehead from constant bruising by a football helmet.

hip pointer: an injury at the front point of the hip, usually a tear of the muscle from the bone, sometimes with a small fracture of the bone.

hitting the wall: suddenly running out of steam in the final miles of a marathon.

horse kiss: a large black-and-blue mark on the side of the thigh from a kick, usually in soccer.

jammed joint: a sprain of the middle joint of a finger.

jersey finger: a rupture of the tendon at the end of the finger, caused by catching the finger on an opponent's jersey or shoulder pad in football.

jock itch: a rash and raw, itchy inflammation in the groin, frequently related to a fungus infection.

jumper's ankle: pain in the front of the ankle from repeated jumping.

jumper's knee: a pain at the base of the kneecap from excessive jumping in basketball and other jumping sports.

knock-down shoulder: a partial shoulder separation.

lifter's shoulder: an acute, sometimes chronic, pain in the front of the shoulder caused by a strain or tear in the ligaments from excessive bench-lifting of heavy weights.

lineman's back: a backache caused by the back being bent forcefully backwards during blocking in football.

Little League elbow: an injury where the muscles and tendons are connected at the bone on the inner or outer side of the elbow. A baseball pitcher's injury related to throwing curve balls.

mallet finger: see *baseball finger*.

oscar: slang term for Osgood-Schlatter's knee, a painful knee condition.

pitcher's arm: soreness from the shoulder to the elbow caused by excessive throwing.

runner's knee: discomfort in the outer side of the knee along the edge of the kneecap or below the knee.

shoulder shift: chronic condition in which the shoulder shifts out of place and back almost instantaneously.

skater's bump: a bump on the front of the ankle or just above it, caused by the skate.

skier's thumb: a ligament tear or fracture on the inner side of the thumb, caused when the thumb is caught in the ski-pole strap during a fall.

soccer foot: swelling of the long tendon of the big toe, causing pain on the instep or top of the foot.

soccer toe: acute pain at the base or top of the big toe from constant kicking. May be accompanied by swelling and a callus.

spearing: using the helmet as a battering ram to attack an opponent in football. A dangerous maneuver that has been outlawed in high-school and college football.

stick blocking: see *spearing*.

stinger: see *burner*.

stitch: a sudden muscle cramp, usually at one's side just below the ribs.

surfer's foot: a thick callus on top of the foot from friction against the surfboard.

swimmer's ear: an infection of the inner canal of the ear.

swimmer's shoulder: pain in the shoulder caused by excessive strain in swimming.

tennis elbow: pain on the outer point of the elbow related to excessive gripping of the racquet.

tennis toe: see *black toe*.

turf toe: a painful toe from pushing off on artificial turf; can lead to arthritis.

wrestler's separation: partial shoulder separation at the sternoclavicular joint.

wry neck: an acute injury in which the neck is bent over and can't be straightened up without pain.

C

Resources on Sports Injuries and Safety

♦

Amateur Athletic Union
    3400 West 86th Street
    Indianapolis, IN 46268
    317/872-2900

American Academy of Pediatricians
    Committee on Sports Medicine
    141 North West Point Boulevard
    Elk Grove Village, IL 60009
    312/228-5005

American Alliance for Health, Physical Education, Recreation, and Dance
    900 Association Drive
    Reston, VA 22091
    703/476-3400

American College of Sports Medicine
    P.O. Box 1440
    Indianapolis, IN 46206
    317/637-9200

American Orthopedic Society for Sports Medicine
    2250 East Deveon Avenue, Suite 115
    Des Plaines, IL 60018
    708/803-8700

American Osteopathic Academy of Sports Medicine
1551 N.W. 54th Street, Suite 200
Seattle, WA 98107
206/782-3383

American Physical Therapy Association
111 North Fairfax Street
Alexandria, VA 22314
703/684-2782

Consumer Product Safety Commission
5401 Westband Avenue
Washington, DC 20207
301/504-0580

National Athletic Trainers Association
2952 Stemmons Freeway
Dallas, TX 75247
214/637-6282

National Federation of State High School Associations
11724 Plaza Circle
Box 20626
Kansas City, MO 64195
816/464-5400

National Operating Committee on Standards for Athletic Equipment (NOCSAE)
11724 Plaza Circle
P.O. Box 20626
Kansas City, MO 64195
816/464-5470

National Safety Council
444 North Michigan Avenue
Chicago, IL 60611
800/621-7619

National Youth Sports Foundation for the Prevention of Sports Injuries
10 Meredith Circle
Needham, MA 02192
617/449-2499

United States Olympic Committee
Sports Medicine
1750 East Boulder Street
Colorado Springs, CO 80909
719/632-5551

D

Resources on Specific Sports

◆

Baseball

Little League International, Inc.
P.O. Box 3485
Williamsport, PA 17701
717/326-1921

Babe Ruth Baseball
P.O. Box 5000
1770 Brunswick Avenue
Trenton, NJ 08630
609/695-1434

Basketball

USA Basketball
1750 East Boulder Street
Colorado Springs, CO 80909
719/632-7687

Cycling

United States Cycling Federation
1750 East Boulder Street
Colorado Springs, CO 80909
719/632-5551

Dance

National Dance Association
1900 Association Drive
Reston, VA 22091
703/476-3490

Equestrian Sports

American Horse Show Association
220 East 42nd Street
New York, NY 10017
212/972-2472

Fencing

United States Fencing Association
1790 East Boulder Street
Colorado Springs, CO 80909
719/632-5551

Field Hockey

United States Field Hockey Association
1750 East Boulder Street
Colorado Springs, CO 80909
719/632-5551

Football

Pop Warner Football
1315 Walnut Street, Suite 1632
Philadelphia, PA 19107
215/735-1450

Golf

American Junior Golf Association
2415 Steeplechase Lane
Roswell, GA 30076
404/998-4653

Gymnastics

Young American Gymnasts
9755 North Conant Street
Kansas City, MO 64153

Hockey

Amateur Hockey Association of the United States
2997 Bradmore Valley Road
Colorado Springs, CO 80906
719/578-4990

Lacrosse

U.S. Women's Lacrosse Association
45 Maple Avenue
Hamilton, NY 13346
315/824-8661

Lacrosse Foundation, Inc.
Newton H. White Athletic Center
Baltimore, MD 21218
301/235-6882

Skating

United States Figure Skating Association
20 First Street
Colorado Springs, CO 80906
719/635-5200

Skiing

United States Skiing Educational Foundation
P.O. Box 100
Park City, UT 84060
801/649-9090

Soccer

United States Soccer Federation
1750 East Boulder Street
Colorado Springs, CO 80909
719/578-4662

United States Youth Soccer Association
1835 Union Avenue, Suite 190
Memphis, TN 38104
800/476-2237

Softball

Amateur Softball Association of America
2801 N.E. 50th Street
Oklahoma City, OK 73111
405/424-5266

Squash and Racquetball

United States Squash and Racquet Association
P.O. Box 1216
23 Cynwyd Road
Bala-Cynwyd, PA 19004
215/667-4006

Swimming

United States Swimming, Inc.
1750 East Boulder Street
Colorado Springs, CO 80909
719/578-4578

AAU USA Junior Olympics
3400 West 86th Street
Indianapolis, IN 46268
317/872-2900

Tennis

United States Tennis Association
707 Alexander Road
Princeton, NJ 08540
609/452-2580

Track and Field

A T Congress
P.O. Box 120
Indianapolis, IN 46206
317/261-0500

Volleyball

United States Volleyball Association
1750 East Boulder Street
Colorado Springs, CO 80909
719/632-5551

Weight Lifting

National Strength and Conditioning Association
300 Old City Hall Landmark
9160 Street, P.O. Box 81410
Lincoln, NE 68501

Wrestling

SA Wrestling
225 South Academy Boulevard
Colorado Springs, CO 80910
719/597-8333

E

Resources on Young Athletes
with Disability

◆

National Handicapped Sports and Recreation Association
4405 East-West Highway, Suite 603
Bethesda, MD 20814
301/652-7505

National Wheelchair Athletic Association
3595 East Fountain Boulevard
Colorado Springs, CO 80910
719/574-1150

Special Olympics International
1350 New York Avenue, N.W., Suite 500
Washington, DC 20005

United States Association for Blind Athletes
33 North Institute Street, Brown Hall Suite 015
Colorado Springs, CO 80903
719/630-0422

United States Cerebral Palsy Athletic Association
34518 Warren Road, Suite 264
Westland, MI 48185
313/425-8961

F

Resources on Coaching Education

◆

American Coaching Effectiveness Program
P.O. Box 5076
Champaign, IL 61825
217/351-5076

Coaching Association of Canada
1600 Prom. James Naismith Drive
Gloucester, Ontario, Canada K1B SN4
613/748-5624

National Youth Sports Coaches Association
2611 Old Okeechobee Road
West Palm Beach, FL 33409
407/684-1141

Youth Sports Institute
Michigan State University
213 I.M. Sports Circle
East Lansing, MI 48824
517/353-6689

G

Suggested Readings

◆

You may find these books useful for further information about youth sports injuries.

Bergeron, J. D., and H. W. Green. *Coaches Guide to Sports Injuries*. Champaign, IL: Human Kinetics Publishers Inc., 1989.

Clark, N. *The Athlete's Kitchen*. New York: Bantam Books, 1981.

Fox, J. M., and R. McGuire. *Save Your Knees*. New York: Dell Publishing, 1988.

Glover, B., and M. Weisenfeld. *The Injured Runner's Training Handbook*. New York: Viking Penguin Inc., 1985.

Hannaway, P., M.D. *The Asthma Self-Help Book*. Marblehead, MA: Lighthouse Press, 1989.

Magill, R. A., et al. *Children in Sport*. Champaign, IL: Human Kinetics Publishers Inc., 1982.

Martens, R. *Joy and Sadness in Children's Sports*. Champaign, IL: Human Kinetics Publishers Inc., 1978.

Paciorek, M. J., and J. A. Jones. *Sports and Recreation for the Disabled*. Indianapolis: Benchmark Press, 1989.

Peterson, M., and K. Peterson. *Eat to Compete*. Chicago: Year Book Medical Publishers Inc., 1988.

Ryan, A. J., M.D., and R. E. Stephans, Ph.D. *The Dancer's Complete Guide to Health Care and a Long Career*. Chicago: Bonus Books, 1988.

Ryan, A. J., M.D., and F. L. Allman, Jr., M.D. *Sports Medicine*. San Diego: Academic Press, 1989.

Smith, N., M.D., et al. *Handbook for the Young Athlete*. Palo Alto, CA: Bull Publishing Company, 1978.

Southmayd, W., M.D., and M. Hoffman. *Sports Health*. New York: Quick Fox Publishers, 1984.

Voth, H. M., M.D., and G. Nahas, M.D. *How to Save Your Child from Drugs*. Middlebury, VT: Paul S. Erickson, Publisher, 1987.

Index

◆